The Challenged Resident

Aloysius Ochasi

The Challenged Resident

Moral Distress, Moral Disengagement, and Ethical Climate in U.S. Medical Residencies

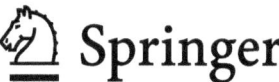 Springer

Aloysius Ochasi
Bioethics and Interdisciplinary Studies
East Carolina University
Greenville, NC, USA

ISBN 978-3-031-71205-0 ISBN 978-3-031-71206-7 (eBook)
https://doi.org/10.1007/978-3-031-71206-7

This Springer imprint is published by the registered company Springer Nature Switzerland AG
The registered company address is: Gewerbestrasse 11, 6330 Cham, Switzerland

If disposing of this product, please recycle the paper.

To my parents of blessed memory, Livinus A. W. and Regina C. Ochasi, whose unconditional love nurtured me and whose guidance instilled in me the importance of education and hard work.

Foreword

Very early in my career, I had the privilege of being invited into what I would characterize as sacred space. The setting I'm referencing is Family Medicine's Morning Report. I recall each morning at 0730, watching the residents file in while one of the interns was always nervously pulling together the case to present to their peers and faculty. And there I was, often standing in the back of a room that doubled as the nurses' break room where, for the next hour, no one outside of this group gathered would enter. It was a room where a discussion of a patient that presented a particular challenge to the team was about to be dissected at a level that is rarely afforded the time in today's healthcare operations. The goal of Morning Report was twofold for these young physicians: (a) learn to provide a concise summary of a patient through a thorough review of organ systems with a precise question for consultation; and (b) learn the art of creating a differential.

Although I had worked with many of the family medicine residents throughout their entire 3-year journey, the idea of being present here, by invitation from residency faculty, always felt a little voyeuristic. I often wondered what the residents thought of an ethicist sitting in Morning Report when it was so obviously physician-focused. Early on, I felt their glances in my direction seemingly asking, "What is he doing here?" though no one ever stated this explicitly. As the months went on, the conversations on tough cases often changed from "What is he doing here?" to "I'm so glad you are here…what do you think?" It is when this question changed, along with the implicit increased level of trust that allowed the question to come forward, that I began to first understand the depths of moral distress and moral disengagement our family medicine residents were experiencing. This is precisely why Aloysius Ochasi's work is so critical for what it means to be a physician.

Ochasi's exploration of moral distress and moral disengagement for residents in the United States (U.S.) began as a prior study in which he examined the causes of moral distress and how that moral distress can lead to moral disengagement. Both can have a detrimental impact on patient care which he illustrates well through a comprehensive review of the literature in other related healthcare fields in chaps. 1 and 2. Leaning on the literature in nursing enables Dr. Ochasi to cover significant terrain and decades of findings on moral distress in clinical practice that can contribute to everything from impact on care to outright exiting from the profession. His exploration of moral disengagement as it relates to moral distress suggests that, when moral distress is at its worst, individuals may "turn off" certain mechanisms that need to be triggered or activated to create optimal care environments. Where such moral disengagement may occur, a host of actions may result that would be characterized as inhumane conduct in the healthcare setting, most specifically dehumanizing the patient or even attributing blame for the disease on the patient him or herself. To determine the extent to which moral distress and moral disengagement may be prevalent early in a physician's career is the critical next step in the literature on moral distress and moral disengagement to which Ochasi directs the field.

In chap. 3, Ochasi takes an important look at healthcare itself in order to better understand whether and, if so, to what extent the organizational climate plays a role in moral distress and moral disengagement. Again, turning to the wealth of literature on these relationships related to nursing practice, Ochasi concludes that an ethical climate "is the single most important factor in explaining nurses' turnover intentions," which he notes early as a well-documented outcome of moral distress. It is not a significant leap, therefore, to suggest that the ethical climate of the healthcare setting in which residents find themselves may present the same troubling factor for physicians. However, unique to residents is the fact that such an outcome may create feelings of being trapped as opposed to outright departure from the field, given the fact that residents are de facto early in their careers as physicians and the extent to which the degree itself does not present many career options outside of fulfilling the requirements to become a physician.

In chap. 4, Ochasi returns to his original quantitative research. His investigation attempts to determine (a) to what extent, if any, does the frequency and intensity of the experience of moral distress predict the propensity for moral disengagement among U.S. residents; and (b) does the perception of the ethical climate of the healthcare environment moderate the predictive relationship? His findings suggest a statistically significant relationship between the frequency and intensity of the experience of moral distress as a predictor of the propensity for moral disengagement among U.S. residents; however, his research does not suggest that the ethical climate of the institution serves to moderate the relationship between the two. The research included 150 resident respondents of which 96 met inclusion criteria from 14 acute care hospitals in the eastern and midwestern United States from a variety of specialties with the exception of surgery and pediatrics.

The value of Ochasi's quantitative analysis on U.S. residents in and of itself is an important contribution to the literature on moral distress and moral disengagement. It is his qualitative research, however, specifically the resident interviews, that struck me as incredibly fertile ground for ongoing research and exploration. Regardless of whether the interviews were of an intern or a more experienced resident, the narratives were often gut-wrenching. Phrases were used to describe incredibly challenging clinical circumstances that, from my perspective, should never be equated with healthcare delivery. To hear a resident recall an experience where they were told, "You are a resident, just shut up and do what your attending says" or, relative to a particularly challenging case, a resident commented that "...I know moral distress is common and occurs daily in residency, but this one was in a league of its own" or in response to feeling powerless in the face of ongoing medical interventions "No one would even listen if I said anything." These interviews alone, as part of Ochasi's qualitative research, should give all in healthcare pause and serve as a call for further exploration of the depth and breadth of the impact of moral distress and moral disengagement in and among U.S. residency programs.

In chap. 6, Ochasi attempts to respond to this call by offering suggestions for leadership of residency programs to continue to work to recognize the problem of moral distress and moral disengagement and the threat they pose to residents, their patients, and the culture of medicine as a whole. To put a finer point on the matter, in chap. 7, Ochasi explores the phenomena of moral distress and moral disengagement through the lens of residency experiences during COVID-19, given that his quantitative and qualitative study concluded just prior to the start of the pandemic in the United States. He rightly notes that understanding the impact of moral distress and moral disengagement outside of these unique and exponentially more challenging circumstances should be a priority for the profession in order to be better prepared for the next global healthcare crisis. Finally, Ochasi ends with a brief review of current recommendations from the literature on what residents may do individually to work through the experience of moral distress in patient care.

I commend Ochasi for his unwillingness to take the wealth of literature on moral distress in nursing and physician practice and simply apply it to medical residency. Ochasi recognizes the unique dimensions of residency programs and applies rigorous quantitative and qualitative analytics to the question of whether and to what extent moral distress may lead to moral disengagement for medical residents. Ochasi's work begins to fill a gap in the critically important work on moral distress by focusing on the experience of medical residents in the United States and will undoubtedly be a significant basis for ongoing research in this important area of healthcare delivery.

Milwaukee, WI   Mark Repenshek

Acknowledgments

I could not have written this book without the support of many individuals. I wish to express my profound appreciation to Mark Repenshek, PhD, for his honest and constructive feedback. His insightful and creative suggestions significantly improved the quality of this work. I thank Helen Bailie, PhD, for her expert guidance and meticulous editing. I owe a debt of gratitude to my professional colleagues: Kirk Mensch, PhD, Peter Clark, SJ, PhD, Marvin Lee, PhD, Rob Danoff, MD, Hebert Patrick, MD, Greg Hassler, PhD, Maria Clay, PhD, and Bege Dauda, PhD. They provided constant inspiration, encouragement, and collaboration. The fraternity and conviviality of my faculty colleagues at the Department of Bioethics and Interdisciplinary Studies at the Brody School of Medicine, East Carolina University, made this an engaging scholarly experience, for which I am grateful. Finally, this book would not have been possible without the support of my family and friends. I am forever grateful to my siblings and their families for being my greatest cheerleaders. I cherish you all.

Introduction

According to the Association of American Colleges, active medical residents in the United States numbered around 144,660 in 2021. These included residents in a wide range of fields such as orthopedic surgery, pediatrics, and emergency medicine. The path to becoming full-time doctors is not an easy one. In the course of their residencies, medical residents face intense pressures that include financial burdens, heavy workloads, and constant evaluations, as well as the knowledge that they bear the responsibility for their patients' health. It is not uncommon for these stressors to result in depression and anxiety, as well as impact the physical well-being of residents, which ultimately can have an effect on the quality of patient care. Moreover, the constant pressure residents experience can lead to three specific phenomena that can have a bearing on their abilities to function effectively within their programs: moral distress, moral disengagement, and how they perceive the ethical climate of the healthcare organizations in which they work.

The first phenomenon, moral distress, has garnered the attention of researchers because it has become a central and dominant issue in healthcare. However, until recently, the medical field has focused on moral distress in relation to nursing and has given less attention to the impact of moral distress on medical residents. The nurse-philosopher Andrew Jameton coined the term "moral distress" in 1984. It is defined as a situation that arises "when one knows the right thing to do, but institutional constraints make it nearly impossible to pursue the right course of action" [1]. For medical residents, this can result in conflicts, such as ones between what a resident knows is the ethically appropriate action when treating a patient and what a patient's surrogate desires. In such instances, a surrogate's insistence on aggressive and ineffective medical treatment for a dying patient rather than transitioning to comfort measures may be a source of moral distress for residents who view such treatment as a violation of the ethical obligation to "do no harm" (nonmaleficence).

The second phenomenon that can impact residents' ability to function effectively within their programs is moral disengagement. Moral disengagement, which falls under the umbrella of social cognitive theory (SCT), refers to the "social cognitive process in which people disengage their internalized moral standards from external immoral behaviors in order to persuade themselves that the deviant behaviors are actually morally permissible" [2]. Moral disengagement and moral distress often are associated loosely, as it is believed that moral distress leads to moral disengagement. Within a hospital setting, morally disengaged health professionals treat patients "less like persons and more like objects," [3] which can impact patient safety and quality of care.

The third phenomenon is the residents' perception of the ethical climate of healthcare organizations. Ethical climate has been defined variously as "those shared perceptions of organizational practices related to ethical decision-making and reflection, and includes issues of power, trust and human interactions within an organization" [4] or the "organizational conditions and practices that affect the way difficult patient care problems, with ethical implications, are discussed and handled" [5]. The ethical climate of healthcare organizations, both positive and negative, plays a crucial role in shaping the behavior of their employees. For instance, a hospital's negative ethical climate can be associated with residents' physical and mental burdens, less time for direct face-to-face care between residents and patients, strained relations with hospital managers and other healthcare professionals, and moral dilemmas related to patient care, among other issues. In contrast, a healthcare organization's positive ethical climate encourages ethical behavior, teamwork, job satisfaction, and retention.

While moral distress and moral disengagement have been linked together loosely in previous studies, there has, in fact, been no empirical verification that they are associated. The paucity of research on this topic has been partly due to the medical establishment's disinclination to admit moral distress and moral disengagement might be outcomes of how medicine has designed its residency programs and the resulting pressures these programs put on medical residents. However, whether or not the medical establishment acknowledges the ethical climate of residency programs leads to moral distress and moral disengagement, what is indisputable is the effect of residents' physical and mental well-being on the care of patients. Moral distress has biological, psychological, and stress-related consequences on medical residents that can lead to ineffective patient healthcare and career dissatisfaction.

What impact does such a discussion have on the health field and why is it important in relation to medical residents? To begin with, it contributes to the knowledge base for healthcare organizations in understanding issues of moral distress, moral disengagement, and the role of the ethical climate among residents. It also may underscore the need for hospital administrators, directors of residency programs, medical faculty, and policymakers to develop appropriate mechanisms to effectively address the interplay between moral distress and moral disengagement among residents. Furthermore, it can provide residents with the appropriate language and frame of reference they need to articulate distressing situations they may have experienced in the past and thought were isolated incidences or simply a part of residency. These phenomena require serious consideration in the healthcare landscape, as it is increasingly acknowledged that moral distress can have "negative and long-lasting effects that can lead healthcare providers to become desensitized to the moral dimensions of their work or even leave their profession" [6].

The Challenged Resident—Moral Distress, Moral Disengagement, and Ethical Climate in U.S. Medical Residencies is based on a prior study I undertook to explore this topic. The study examined not only the causes of moral distress among medical residents but also how it can lead to moral disengagement. In this book, I begin by giving an overview of the scholarship on moral distress experienced by practitioners within the medical establishment and its negative psychological outcomes. Chapter 2 examines how moral distress can lead to moral disengagement and its effect on patients. Chapter 3 looks at the residents' perception of the role of ethical climate on moral distress. In chap. 4, I describe the impetus behind the study that prompted this book and how it was carried out. Chapter 5 reviews the findings of that study to examine more closely the relationship between moral distress and moral disengagement and the role ethical climate plays within the medical establishment. In chap. 6, I summarize the quantitative and qualitative findings of the study. I go on to discuss how these issues were addressed and handled during the recent COVID-19 pandemic in chap. 7, when medical personnel were often stressed, overworked, and apprehensive about getting the virus themselves. Subsequently, in chap. 8, I suggest ways the phenomena of moral distress and moral disengagement can be avoided and what medical residents can do to manage the stresses inherent in navigating the demands of medical training. My hope is that this book will bring awareness to the pressures and stressors medical residents experience that often lead to moral disengagement and, in turn, impact their interactions with their patients. The implementation of strategies I suggest, from the application of new policies to self-care, should result in a more positive working environment that ultimately improves the quality of patient care.

References

1. Jameton A. Dilemmas of moral distress: moral responsibility and nursing practice. WHONNS Clin Issues Perinat Womens Health Nurs. 1993;4(4):542–51. https://pubmed.ncbi.nlm.nih.gov/8220368/.
2. Bandura A. Moral disengagement in the perpetration of inhumanities. Pers Soc Psychol Rev. 1999;3(3):193–209.
3. Haque OS, Waytz A. Dehumanization in medicine: causes, solutions, and functions. Perspect Psychol Sci. 2012;7(2):176–86. https://doi.org/10.1177/1745691611429706.
4. Olson LL. Hospital nurses' perceptions of the ethical climate of their work setting. J Nurs Scholarsh. 1998;30(4):345–9. https://doi.org/10.1111/j.1547-5069.1998.tb01331.x.
5. Hart SE. Hospital ethical climates and registered nurses' turnover intentions. J Nurs Scholarsh. 2005;37(2):173–7. https://doi.org/10.1111/j.1547-5069.2005.00030.x.
6. Hamric AB, Davis WS, Childress MD. Moral distress in health care professionals. Pharos Alpha Omega Alpha Honor Med Soc. 2006;69(1):16–23. https://pubmed.ncbi.nlm.nih.gov/16544460/.

Contents

List of Figures

List of Tables

About the Author

Aloysius Ochasi is an Associate Professor in the Department of Bioethics and Interdisciplinary Studies at the Brody School of Medicine, East Carolina University, North Carolina. He holds dual doctorate degrees in Bioethics and Organizational Leadership. Before joining Brody, he taught bioethics at St. Joseph's University in Philadelphia, Pennsylvania, and leadership courses at the MacArthur School of Leadership, Palm Beach Atlantic University, Florida. As a clinical bioethicist, he has conducted ethics teaching rounds, lectures, and consultations for over 500 medical students, interns, residents, and fellows at 14 acute-care hospitals across four states in the Northeast. Dr. Ochasi has authored book chapters and numerous articles in both national and international bioethics journals. His research interests include moral distress and moral disengagement in healthcare, the role of artificial intelligence in medicine, reusable medical devices in low- and middle-income countries, health equity and access, and organ donation and transplantation.

Chapter 1
The Issue of Moral Distress

Moral distress is a challenging problem for residents and other healthcare workers that can result in negative psychological outcomes and a decrease in job retainment. It can be a direct outcome of the stressors medical residents face during their residencies that may affect not only patient care but also the residents' ability to function effectively within their programs. This chapter gives an overview of the scholarship on moral distress within the medical establishment, which is integral to understanding the relationship between moral distress and moral disengagement, along with ethical climate contributes to this issue. To date, much of the research on this topic has focused on nurses. However, medical residents often face the same pressures other medical personnel experience. In reviewing the literature on moral distress, I extend the discussion to include how the findings can apply to medical residents and include interviews with various residents who relate occurrences during their medical training that led to experiences of moral distress.

Moral Distress

Moral distress occurs when a clinician is unable to act in accordance with their ethical beliefs as a result of external constraints, notably those related to hierarchy or institutional culture. In describing the powerlessness commonly felt by clinicians who experience moral distress, Hamric et al. wrote,

> Moral distress is a real problem … especially in medical students, residents, nurses, respiratory care, and other allied health workers … people who see themselves as involved in morally significant relationships with sick, vulnerable humans, but have little or no power to respond when what is happening appears to be "wrong" [1].

These authors explained that most clinicians, especially nurses and medical residents, are often "caught between" attending physicians and patients and their

© The Author(s), under exclusive license to Springer Nature
Switzerland AG 2024
A. Ochasi, *The Challenged Resident*,
https://doi.org/10.1007/978-3-031-71206-7_1

families. As people who directly interact with their patients and families, residents have the needed information to formulate a care plan, yet the resident might not be consulted during the decision-making process and, at times, may be expected to implement a treatment plan contrary to their ethical beliefs, which can lead to residents experiencing moral distress. Hamric and Blackhall's work reveals that, when caring for dying patients in the ICU, both nurses and physicians often experience moral distress, especially when there is pressure to continue aggressive treatment where it may not be clinically appropriate [2]. This is exemplified in a response a medical resident who took part in my study gave to a situation in which the patient had no chance of recovery but, the parent insisted "everything should be done." The resident described it as feeling as if they were "torturing" the patient, adding, "I would say it was an emotional roller coaster for me. I was angry at the mother and the entire team, including the hospital administration, for letting this patient go through this ordeal." The resident went on to comment that, at times, the moral distress she felt made her physically ill, and there were days when she had to leave the ICU to clear her head.

In his seminal work on moral distress, Jameton categorized the moral and ethical problems medical personnel face in hospitals into three different types: moral uncertainty (when one is unsure what moral principle or value applies or even what the moral problem is); moral dilemmas (when two or more clear moral principles apply, but they support mutually inconsistent courses of action); and moral distress (when "one knows the right thing to do, but institutional constraints make it nearly impossible to pursue the right course of action") [3]. Such constraints or obstacles include medical power structures, institutional policies, supervisory reluctance, lack of time, and legal restrictions, all of which inhibit action on the part of medical practitioners.

Jameton elaborated on the concept of moral distress by distinguishing between two types: initial and reactive moral distress. Initial distress involves "the feelings of frustration, anger, and anxiety people experience when faced with institutional obstacles and conflict with others about values" [3]. During one interview, a medical resident exemplified initial distress when she described a 95-year-old woman who had stage four lung cancer with metastasis to the liver and brain and was admitted to the emergency room with a broken hip. Although she had informed her family and medical personnel that she did not want any aggressive measures applied and the specialists had decided it would be in her best interest not to operate to repair the hip fracture, the family insisted that the operation take place and the cardiologist agreed. Though the patient died the night before surgery, the resident was left with feelings of frustration and guilt that the hospital staff had been prepared to ignore the patient's wishes declaring,

> Even though I made my concerns known to the attending physician, I felt helpless because the odds were stacked against me. It looked like there was not much I could have done. You know, as residents, the chain of command in every team goes through the attending of record.

Here, the resident perceived the patient's wishes were being overruled, which provoked for the resident not only feelings of anger but also of helplessness.

The second type of distress Jameton described, reactive distress, is "the distress that people feel when they do not act upon their initial distress" [3]. In the example describing the continued treatment of the 95-year-old patient, the resident reported how, for a long time afterward, "I felt as if I did not speak up enough to challenge the decisions of the family, and this made me angry"—perhaps illustrating how residents might feel when they have no control over a situation and thus exhibiting reactive distress.

Judith M. Wilkinson, who studied how nurses react to moral distress, built on Jameton's description by defining moral distress as "the psychological disequilibrium, and negative feeling state experienced when a person makes a moral decision but does not follow through by performing the moral behavior indicated by that decision" [4]. Wilkinson developed a moral distress model in an interview-related study with 24 Intensive Care Unit (ICU) nurses based on Jameton's definition of moral distress. The interview responses led to the generation of conceptual categories of moral distress, including cognitive, situational, feeling, and action dimensions. These categories became known as the indicators of moral distress that either "contribute to or are influenced by moral distress" [4]. The morally distressing cases varied among the participants, but the study categorized predominant ones as unnecessary prolongation of life and aggressive treatment, the continuation of unnecessary tests and procedures, physicians' inadequate or incompetent treatment, and lying to patients. Contextual constraints the study participants identified were both external and internal. The external constraints that prevent nurses from doing the right thing include physicians, nurse administrators, hospital policies, and laws or lawsuits, while the internal constraints align with "being socialized to follow orders, futility of past actions, fear of losing their jobs, self-doubt, and lack of courage" [4]. It is necessary to point out that the internal constraints mentioned in Wilkinson's study, such as fear of losing jobs and lack of courage, relate more to an ethical climate, which I discuss later in this chapter. The internal factors the perception of an ethical climate create are not, by definition, aspects of moral distress as Jameton put forth.

Wilkinson's concept of moral distress varies from Jameton's in that, in her view, moral distress encapsulates both the medical professional's experience and the effect on patient care. The healthcare professional experiencing this moral distress may devise coping mechanisms, such as patient avoidance or compensation, which ultimately affects patient care. A significant observation of Wilkinson's is that moral distress does not occur automatically just because a particular case happens; rather, it requires a conflict between the nurse's belief system and elements of that case [4]. For example, in cases of cardio-pulmonary resuscitation (CPR) for a patient, some nurses might suffer moral distress if CPR was performed, while others might suffer moral distress if it was not, depending on their beliefs about quality of life, killing, and letting a person die. Wilkinson observed nurses who held similar values as the physicians and the hospital where they were employed seemed to suffer fewer instances of moral distress. Wilkinson also found the effects of moral distress on the nurses were systemic and affected their entire being. Some of the effects include loss of self-worth, impact on personal relationships, feelings of depression, nightmares, and physical symptoms of diarrhea, heart palpitations, and headaches [4].

When moral distress creates a psychological disequilibrium, coping behaviors are paramount for enabling nurses to make moral decisions and act in the patient's best interests. According to Wilkinson, the two most common successful coping behaviors for nurses who participated in her study were to deny responsibility for the situation or for their immoral/unethical action and to believe they could exert some control and have some effect on patient care [4]. In essence, moral distress has a dual impact on both nurse and patient care. The nurses reported the frustrations, anger, and guilt emanating from moral distress often made them avoid the patients and even leave the nursing profession.

Some of the issues that arose from Wilkinson's studies are similar to those medical residents encounter, such as unnecessary prolongation of life and aggressive treatment, the continuation of unnecessary tests and procedures, physicians' inadequate or incompetent treatment, and lying to patients. Similarly to nurses, medical residents are faced with external constraints—from physicians, hospital policies, or the threat of lawsuits—that prevent them from doing what they think is in the patient's best interest. The internal constraints medical residents experience align with "being socialized to follow orders, futility of past actions, fear of losing their jobs, self-doubt, and lack of courage" [4].

For Wilkinson, moral distress does not occur automatically because of a particular case; rather, it requires a conflict between the practitioner's belief system and elements of that case [4]. For instance, one medical resident was troubled that the prognosis for one patient was being kept from her:

> Being forced by my attending to engage in calculated deception of not discussing the patient's prognosis was unnerving. It was unconscionable. I felt like I was an accomplice. This was not even a case of giving false hope because that would entail letting the patient know the prognosis before giving them false hope. This was a case of deceit. This violated her right to know her diagnosis and prognosis as a human being.

The resident added that, in feeling part of a conspiracy, "my instinct is withdrawal and avoidance of the unpleasant environment". In some cases, the physiological and emotional effects can lead to medical residents leaving the field of medicine altogether.

Although these studies illustrate the importance of the concept of moral distress, what also becomes apparent is the lack of consistency, consensus, and conceptual clarity concerning the definition of moral distress. For Webster and Baylis, moral distress occurs when

> one fails to pursue what one believes to be the right course of action (or fails to do so to one's satisfaction) for one or more of the following reasons: an error in judgment, some personal failing (for example, a weakness or crimp in one's character such as a pattern of "systemic avoidance"), or other circumstances truly beyond one's control [5].

Recall that, for Jameton, moral distress occurs "when one knows the right thing to do, but institutional constraints make it nearly impossible to pursue the right course of action" [3]. Webster and Baylis's definition highlights the external constraints instrumental to moral distress. However, unlike Jameton, Baylis and Webster put the onus on the individual's inability to act squarely on the individual instead of on the systemic failures that contribute to moral distress (qtd. in Varcoe et al.) [6]. In this way, moral constraints might be construed as personal failings external to the individual experiencing the distress. Repenshek argues that Jameton's definition of moral distress has remained uncritically examined because the context of how moral distress arises (i.e., anger, frustration, powerlessness, and so on) has been appropriated as its definition. He opined the vast majority of literature on moral distress may "truly be measuring contexts wherein moral distress may arise, rather than truly measuring the concept of moral distress" [7].

Despite these inconsistencies, there are some who believe moral distress has the potential to foster positive outcomes. For instance, experiences of moral distress may encourage critical reflection and exploration of moral wrongdoing, promote self-reflective practice, and engender empathy, compassion, and moral sensitivity among practitioners. Individuals who experience moral distress may adopt coping mechanisms and add personal moral insight to their engagements. Another outcome may be to encourage support networks and multidisciplinary collaboration to uncover attitudes and values, ultimately leading to stronger collegial relationships. Nonetheless, the real impact of moral distress may be so disproportionately burdensome to suggest any positive outcomes are justifiable. Turning to empirical research on moral distress in nursing may offer some clarity on this question.

Empirical Research on Moral Distress Among Nurses

Many of the factors that cause moral distress in nurses are the same as those medical residents experience and, in fact, can apply to other medical personnel. For example, Rice et al. conducted a cross-sectional study with 260 medical and surgical nurses to determine the prevalence and contributing factors of moral distress using the moral distress scale (MDS) Hamric et al. developed [8]. The findings showed moral distress is uniformly high in situations related to "physician practice, nursing practice, institutional factors, futile care, deception, and euthanasia" [8]. Distressing situations associated with futile care, deceptions, and caring for oncology and transplant patients were exceptionally high, and nursing experience exacerbated the intensity and frequency of moral distress.

In their study, Corley et al. suggested nurses have values and feel moral responsibility, but because of institutional constraints, their "values do not consistently direct their behavior" [9]. The institutional constraints that impede individual responsibility, acting in the patient's best interest, and truth-telling contribute to causing moral distress among nurses. In fact, 15% of nurses surveyed had left their previous positions due to moral distress. In Corley's theory of nurse moral distress, two contexts of moral distress are addressed: the internal context, namely nurses' psychological responses, and the external context, namely the work environment

[10]. In addition, Corley discussed the relationship between moral distress and other moral concepts that precede or follow moral distress, such as moral integrity, moral sensitivity, moral commitment, moral competency, moral imagination, moral certainty, moral conflict, moral outrage, moral courage, moral heroism, and moral behavior (moral agency). Corley highlighted the act of nursing as a moral endeavor that is fundamentally ethical. Therefore, nurses suffer moral distress when their ethics-laden professional goals are impeded [10]. While Corley's study uncovered some of the causes and effects of moral distress, there is still a need to reemphasize that the working definition of moral distress by Jameton involves institutional and external constraints different from Corley's conceptualization of the phenomenon.

Following the effects of moral distress, residents, nurses, and other healthcare practitioners may continue to experience guilt, powerlessness, and depression in the form of moral residue. Moral residue refers to the feelings that linger after a morally distressing situation has passed. Epstein and Hamric proposed the crescendo effect model to describe the interrelationship between moral distress and moral residue. After each morally distressing situation, some moral residues remain, forming a new baseline for moral distress. Repeated increase in both moral distress and moral residue gives rise to higher crescendos. Thus, the crescendo of moral residue is an amalgam of a healthcare practitioner's unresolved moral distress, which is most damaging in the future [11]. This study shows the crescendo effect is multidisciplinary and goes beyond nurses to incorporate physicians.

Epstein and Delgado showed repeated exposure to moral distress can devastate one's moral sensitivity to problematic and challenging clinical situations and one's career. The lingering effects of moral distress leave moral residue even after the distressing situation resolves, but the moral distress crescendo occurs as a clinical situation unfolds [12]. The authors extrapolated three potential consequences of moral distress and moral residue: moral numbness to ethically challenging situations, engaging in different ways of conscientiously objecting to the trajectory of the situation, and burnout [12]. The section below reviews how empirical studies on moral distress and nurses extend to other healthcare workers.

Moral Distress Among Other Healthcare Professionals

As previously noted, while overwhelmingly studies on moral distress have been conducted in nursing, researchers have recently extended them to other healthcare specialties. Hamric et al. outlined the clinical situations and internal and external factors responsible for moral distress among healthcare professionals in general. Their study provided evidence that indicates feelings of powerlessness are also common in clinicians who experience moral distress:

> Moral distress is a real problem … especially in medical students, residents, nurses, respiratory care and other allied health workers … people who see themselves as involved in morally significant relationships with sick, vulnerable humans, but have little or no power to respond when what is happening appears to be "wrong" [1].

They explained that most clinicians, especially nurses and medical residents, are caught between attending physicians and patients and their families. As people who interact with the patients, residents know them and their families well and gather the needed information to formulate a care plan. Moral distress may occur when clinicians are not consulted during the decision-making process and are expected to implement a treatment plan contrary to their ethical beliefs.

Hamric and Blackhall, in examining the nurse-physician perspective of moral distress in relation to caring for dying patients in the ICU, stated that while both experience moral distress, especially with the pressure to continue aggressive treatment where it is not clinically appropriate, registered nurses (RNs) experience more moral distress and lower collaboration in comparison to physicians [2]. They also perceived the ethical climate to be more negative and "were less satisfied with the quality of care provided on their units than were physicians" [2]. The study underscored a common ground that demonstrates the reality of moral distress and served as a starting point for discussions on mitigating its negative effects. It is essential to point out that not every example of clinically inappropriate medical intervention may be an experience of moral distress based on Jameton's definition of moral distress. There has to be the presence of an institutional pressure or constraint against doing what one believes to be true to meet Jameton's criteria.

Hamric gave an overview of the empirical research that has helped identify some of the root causes of moral distress that include: (a) the factors internal to the caregiver (perceived powerlessness and lack of knowledge of alternatives or the full situation); (b) the external factors in the situation (institutional constraints, such as inadequate staffing, lack of administrative support, and incompetent caregivers); and (c) the clinical situations (futile treatment, aggressive treatment not in the patient's best interest, inadequate informed consent, and lack of truth-telling, such as giving false hope) [13]. These studies highlight the reality of moral distress because "it is so powerful and so destructive to the moral agency and integrity of healthcare providers" [13]. Hamric concluded moral distress can compromise the core values or duties of providers, which cascade over time into moral desensitization or exit from the profession [13]. The importance of Hamric's analysis is that it gives a synopsis of the variety of situations that could cause moral distress.

Garros, in analyzing the effects of moral distress in the everyday life of an intensivist, affirmed intra-team discordance—such as power imbalances, silencing, professional tribalism, and lack of trust in existing mechanisms for ethical dialogue and patient management—can affect and heighten moral distress among pediatric intensive care (PICU) clinicians [14]. Evidence also indicates the intensity of moral distress varies according to two factors: personal moral sensitivity and the moral climate of the organization [14]. In addition, Austin suggested that healthcare environments should support clinicians' moral agency rather than diminish it, as institutional intolerance of dissent "places not only health professionals at greater risk of moral distress, but endangers the well-being of patients, families, and the public" [15]. Medicine is a moral enterprise and healthcare environments should become moral communities instead of simulated marketplaces. Austin concluded healthcare reforms, which undermine the efficacy of health professionals and jeopardize the ethical engagement of those in their care, exacerbate moral distress [15].

Kalvemark et al., in a Sweden-based study of moral distress in a multidisciplinary context, revealed two findings. First, all categories of health staff (physicians, nurses, auxiliary nurses, and medical secretaries) they interviewed, who worked in both hospital clinics and pharmacies, experienced moral distress. Second, moral distress occurs due to institutional constraints preventing the health staff from acting on their moral considerations, which is the traditional definition of moral distress, as well as when the staff members "do follow their moral decisions, but in doing so, they clash with, e.g., legal regulations" [16]. Kalvemark et al. concluded moral distress must focus more on the context of ethical dilemmas than the overwhelming preoccupation with the individual healthcare provider and her subjective moral convictions [16].

In a study of moral distress among Norwegian doctors, Forde and Aasland revealed limited resources and legal regulations cause ethical dilemmas for physicians and induce moral distress. The majority of the physicians (66% of the study sample) experienced distress "related to long waiting lists for treatment and to impaired patient care due to time constraints" [17]. The study concluded moral distress varies with specialty and gender: female physicians experienced more moral distress than their male counterparts. It also found physicians violate their professional self-image, moral standards, and identity as moral agents when they act against their consciences, especially when there is an inadequate workplace mechanism for addressing ethical dilemmas, thereby underscoring the presence of institutional constraints as obstacles to doing what the clinician feels is right [17].

In a study conducted in eight medical-surgical ICUs in the north of Italy to test if the Italian Moral Distress Scale-Revised is a valid and reliable instrument to assess moral distress among critical care clinicians, Lamiani et al. found good reliability in the following four factors when measuring moral distress: futile care, poor teamwork, deceptive communication, and ethical misconduct. Nurses scored higher on futile care than physicians, while physicians scored higher on deceptive communication than nurses. Moral distress was higher for clinicians considering giving up their position. The study further underscored the commonalities of moral distress among health professionals across different cultures [18]. Similarly, in a systematic review of 17 empirical studies, Lamiani et al. revealed moral distress correlates with the following: organizational environment (poor ethical climate and collaboration), professional attitudes (low work satisfaction and engagement), and psychological characteristics (low psychological empowerment and autonomy). They explained that the negative consequences of moral distress affect clinicians' well-being and job retention and jeopardize the quality of care provided to patients [18]. The study supports the claim that health professionals from different specialties experience moral distress.

Rushton et al. examined moral distress among palliative care clinicians and affirmed unmodulated moral distress has the propensity to induce self-focused behaviors, including "avoidance, abandonment, and/or numbing; or resulting in unregulated moral outrage, burnout, or acute secondary stress" [19]. This underscores the claim that moral distress occurs in multidisciplinary clinical situations where clinicians feel "loss of control, stress, discontent, and disheartenment" [19]. These clinicians' negative feelings may affect the type of care their patients receive.

Finally, Abbasi et al. (2014) demonstrated that Iranian physicians showed a moderate level of moral distress when confronted with ethically perplexing situations: "Pediatricians and emergency specialists showed the minimum and maximum mean of composite score of moral distress respectively" [20]. Pediatric wards had the lowest moral distress frequency and the highest moral distress intensity, while emergency wards had the highest moral distress frequency and lowest moral distress intensity. They highlighted moral distress among clinicians does not stem merely from internal constraints, such as self-doubt, fear, anxiety, or lack of confidence, but also from external constraints such as legal, financial, and cross-sectoral policies, in addition to a lack of communication between treatment team members, all of which contribute to moral distress among physicians. They also observed that the moral/ethical atmosphere of the different hospital wards plays a considerable influence on the frequency and intensity of moral distress: "The more positive perception of individual of the moral atmosphere, the less moral distress level develops" [20]. The study showed moral distress was lower among physicians who participated in medical ethics training courses than among those who did not. It is crucial to point out that the internal constraints mentioned in the study align more with the ethical climate. The external constraints, such as legal and financial policies, contribute to moral distress in light of Jameton's definition of the concept.

The review of literature highlights the external and internal constraints that lead to medical personnel experiencing moral distress. Moreover, it emphasizes the effect of the moral/ethical climate of a hospital on personnel's well-being and job retention. The following section reviews studies on moral distress among medical students and residents.

Moral Distress and Medical Residents

Moral distress in medical education begins for medical students during clinical rotations even before they graduate into residency. Wiggleton et al. found during clinical rotation medical students had a strong desire to do what was right and in the patient's best interest, but they often were not able to do so because of systems of care, the hierarchy of medical education, and conflicts with the patients' own values and wishes [21]. The morally distressing situations continue into residency such that, to withstand the pressures brought on by feelings of medical distress, residents and house staff have to develop coping mechanisms such as avoiding patients, pursuing less morally distressing subspecialty careers (rheumatology), practicing moral disengagement, blunting, feeling denial, and using gallows humor [22]. For example, in the case of the parent of the premature neonate with severe neurological problems who insisted that everything should be done for her son, the resident commented, "I became numb. ... I built brick walls around my emotions and developed a thick skin."

Other ethical dilemmas can lead to moral distress for residents. For surgical residents, in particular, the ethical dilemmas include not informing patients about their role, circumstances surrounding the disclosure of intraoperative errors, and dynamics in certain teaching circumstances [23]. This can underscore the feeling of powerlessness among residents when they cannot change certain situations due to institutional constraints and their place in the hierarchy of the care team. In many situations, residents practice under the supervision of an attending physician and feel powerless to challenge their authority.

In the case of pediatric care, residents can experience moral distress due to the following: inexperience and their place in the hierarchy of the medical care team and disagreements with senior staff [24]. While residents working in pediatrics cope with these issues as their residency progresses, they do "not always have opportunities to discuss their concerns in an open and safe forum" [24] which is symptomatic of an institutional culture that either does not recognize the enormity of the problem or pretends it has no impact on residents.

Internal medicine residents may experience significant moral distress when they feel obligated to offer ineffective (futile) treatments at the end of life, as in the example of the elderly patient who received aggressive treatment, though there was no hope of recovery. As a coping mechanism, some of them "develop detached and dehumanizing attitudes towards patients ... which may contribute to a loss of empathy" [25]. Negative consequences of their experiences included burnout, emotional exhaustion, lack of job satisfaction, poor self-image, diminished psychological and physical well-being, and thoughts of quitting. The findings showed residents are more vulnerable to moral distress than physicians because "they are subordinate but on the front line, which reinforces a perceived powerlessness to act as independent moral agents, against treatments that they believe may do more harm than good" [25].

A thorough review of the research shows the common root causes of moral distress are clinical, organizational, interpersonal, and personal. The studies showed moral distress negatively impacts healthcare professionals, patients, and their families. The biological and psychological consequences of moral distress on healthcare professionals revolve around burnout, powerlessness, job satisfaction, and low retention. Even though empirical research on moral distress among medical students and residents is not as extensive as in the nursing profession, the evidence in the literature reviewed supports the claim that moral distress exists among medical students and residents.

The literature also revealed the negative consequences related to moral distress for residents, which include burnout and depersonalization [26]; self-doubt, fear, anxiety, and lack of confidence [20]; dehumanizing attitudes toward patients, loss of empathy, burnout, emotional exhaustion, lack of job satisfaction, poor self-image, diminished psychological and physical well-being, and thoughts of quitting, [25] moral angst and feelings of helplessness, [23] avoidance of patients, moral disengagement, blunting, denial, and use of gallows humor [22]. The list is indeed long. Some of the negative consequences of moral distress, such as detachment, loss of empathy, depersonalization, moral numbness, blunting, and denial, have been loosely associated with moral disengagement. Yet, little is known empirically if these consequences of moral distress for residents turn to moral disengagement. The next chapter explores the concept of moral disengagement with particular emphasis on whether and to what extent there exists a relationship between moral disengagement and moral distress.

References

1. Hamric AB, Davis WS, Childress MD. Moral distress in health care professionals. Pharos. 2006;69(1):16–23. https://pubmed.ncbi.nlm.nih.gov/16544460/.
2. Hamric AB, Blackhall LJ. Nurse-physician perspectives on the care of dying patients in intensive care units: collaboration, moral distress, and ethical climate. Crit Care Med. 2007;35(2):422–9. https://doi.org/10.1097/01.CCM.0000254722.50608.2D.
3. Jameton A. Dilemmas of moral distress: moral responsibility and nursing practice. AWHONNs Clin Issues Perinat Womens Health Nurs. 1993;4(4):542–51. https://pubmed.ncbi.nlm.nih.gov/8220368/.
4. Wilkinson JM. Moral distress in nursing practice: experience and effect. Nurs Forum. 1988;23(1):16–29. https://pubmed.ncbi.nlm.nih.gov/3454003/.
5. Webster GC, Baylis FE. Moral residue. In: Rubin SB, Zoloth L, editors. Margin of error: the ethics of mistakes in the practice of medicine; 2000.
6. Varcoe C, Pauly B, Webster G, Storch J. Moral distress: tensions as springboards for action. HEC Forum. 2012;24(1):51–62. https://doi.org/10.1007/s10730-012-9180-2.
7. Repenshek M. Moral distress: inability to act or discomfort with moral subjectivity? Nurs Ethics. 2009;16(6):734–42. https://pubmed.ncbi.nlm.nih.gov/19889914/.
8. Rice EM, Rady MY, Hamric A, Verheijde JL, Pendergast DK. Determinants of moral distress in medical and surgical nurses at an adult acute tertiary care hospital. J Nurs Manag. 2008;16(3):360–73.
9. Corley MC, Minick P, Elswick RK, Jacobs M. Nurse moral distress and ethical work environment. Nurs Ethics. 2005;12(4):381–90. https://doi.org/10.1191/0969733005ne809oa.
10. Corley MC. Nurse moral distress: a proposed theory and research agenda. Nurs Ethics. 2002;9(6):636–50. https://doi.org/10.1191/0969733002ne557oa.
11. Epstein EG, Hamric AB. Moral distress, moral residue, and the crescendo effect. J Clin Ethics. 2009;20(4):330–42. https://pubmed.ncbi.nlm.nih.gov/20120853/.
12. Epstein EG, Delgado S. Understanding and addressing moral distress. Online J Issues Nurs. 2010;15(3):1B. https://doi.org/10.3912/OJIN.Vol15No03Man01.
13. Hamric AB. Empirical research on moral distress: Issues, challenges, and opportunities. HEC Forum. 2012;24(1):39–49. https://doi.org/10.1007/s10730-012-9177-x.
14. Garros D. Moral distress in the everyday life of an intensivist. Front Pediatr. 2016;4(91):1–4. https://doi.org/10.3389/fped.2016.00091.
15. Austin W. Moral distress and the contemporary plight of health professionals. HEC Forum. 2012;24:27–38.
16. Kalvemark S, Hoglund AT, Hansson MG, Westerholm P, Arnetz B. Living with conflicts—ethical dilemmas and moral distress in the health care system. Soc Sci Med. 2004;58(6):1075–84. https://doi.org/10.1016/s0277-9536(03)00279-x.
17. Forde R, Aasland OG. Moral distress among Norwegian doctors. J Med Ethics. 2008;34(7):521–5. https://doi.org/10.1136/jme.2007.021246.
18. Lamiani G, Setti I, Barlascini L, Vegni E, Argentero P. Measuring moral distress among critical care clinicians: validation and psychometric properties of the Italian moral distress scale-revised. J Crit Care Med. 2017;45(3):430–7. https://doi.org/10.1097/CCM.0000000000002187.

19. Rushton CH, Kaszniak AW, Halifax JS. A framework for understanding moral distress among palliative care clinicians. J Palliat Med. 2013;16(9):1074–9. https://doi.org/10.1089/jpm.2012.0490.

20. Abbasi M, Nejadsarvari N, Kiani M, Borhani F, Bazmi S, Tavaokkoli SN, Rasouli H. Moral distress in physicians practicing in hospitals affiliated to medical sciences universities. Iran Red Crescent Med J. 2014;16(10):e18797. https://doi.org/10.5812/ircmj.18797.

21. Wiggleton C, Petrusa E, Loomis K, Tarpley J, Tarpley M, O'Gorman ML, Miller B. Medical students' experiences of moral distress: development of a web-based survey. Acad Med. 2010;85(1):111–7. https://doi.org/10.1097/ACM.0b013e3181c4782b.

22. Berger JT. Moral distress in medical education and training. J Gen Intern Med. 2013;29(2):395–8. https://doi.org/10.1007/s11606-013-2665-0.

23. Knifed E, Goyal A, Bernstein M. Moral angst for surgical residents: a qualitative study. Am J Surg. 2010;199(4):571–6. https://doi.org/10.1016/j.amjsurg.2009.04.007.

24. Hilliard RI, Harrison C, Madden S. Ethical conflicts and moral distress experienced by paediatric residents during their training. Paediatr Child Health. 2007;12(1):29–35. https://doi.org/10.1093/pch/12.1.29.

25. Dzeng E, Colaianni A, Roland M, Levine D, Kelly MP, Barclay S, Smith TJ. Moral distress among American physician trainees regarding futile treatments at the end of life: a qualitative study. J Gen Intern Med. 2016;31(1):93–9. https://doi.org/10.1007/s11606-015-3505-1.

26. Sajjadi S, Norena M, Wong H, Dodek P. Moral distress and burnout in internal medicine residents. Can Med Educ J. 2017;8(1):e36–43.

Chapter 2
Experiencing Moral Disengagement

Moral disengagement is a concept in social psychology that falls under the umbrella of social cognitive theory (SCT). Social cognitive theory "adopts an interactionist perspective to morality in which moral actions are the products of the reciprocal interplay of personal and social influences" [1]. In SCT, moral reasoning (the process of determining right or wrong in a given situation) is translated into action via self-regulation (the capacity individuals inherently possess to exercise some control over their thought processes, motivation, affect, and action) and control mechanisms anchored in moral standards and self-sanctions by which moral agency is exercised.

Bandura explained individuals as self-regulating agents intentionally influence their functioning and life circumstances. Through this inherent self-regulatory process, people conform and evaluate their actions based on their moral standards (proactive exercise of moral agency) and avoid behaving in ways that violate these standards (an inhibitive form of moral agency) because such moral standard violations would bring self-condemnation [1].

Similarly, self-sanctions are penalties in the form of moral pressure that ensures conformity with one's moral standards. Moral agency or moral self (an individual's ability to make moral judgments with reference to some notion of right and wrong and to be held accountable for these actions) is rooted in an extensive sociocognitive self-theory that encapsulates self-organizing, proactive, self-reflective, and self-regulatory mechanisms [1]. In other words, people conform and evaluate their actions based on their moral standards through this self-regulatory process. These inherent self-referent processes furnish the motivation and cognitively regulate moral conduct. As moral agents, individuals have the ability to freely and constantly exert self-influence on their behavior, whether proactively or by inhibiting their own actions, both of which are aspects of the exercise of moral agency.

The first aspect, the proactive exercise of moral agency, manifests by behaving humanely (nonviolation of the moral standards), while the second aspect, inhibitive form, comes from refraining from engaging in inhumane behavior. The exercise of

A. Ochasi, *The Challenged Resident*,
https://doi.org/10.1007/978-3-031-71206-7_2

this dual nature of morality explains why people do benevolent deeds and refrain from engaging in harmful behaviors. According to SCT, humane behavior incorporates a strong sense of self and social obligation that prevents individuals from acting in a way others perceive to be immoral, even against high personal costs. This explains how individuals with self-worth, principles, and values can sacrifice their self-interest and submit to prolonged maltreatment rather than do what they consider to be morally wrong. In these circumstances, the inability to do what is morally right would bring self-condemnation. A form of morality where a person carries out positive actions and avoids negative actions is known as higher-order morality [2].

People appropriate moral standards during the process of socialization. In the course of socialization, when people observe certain behaviors and the consequences of such behaviors, positive or negative, their replication of these actions shape and guide their subsequent behaviors [3]. Four core properties of human agency are

- Intentionality: the ability to form intentions that include action plans and strategies for actualizing them;
- Forethought: the temporal extension of agency that cognitively visualizes the future and makes it present, as current guides and motivators of behavior;
- Self-reactiveness: the ability to design specific courses of action and to self-motivate and regulate their execution;
- Self-reflectiveness: the ability to deploy self-awareness to evaluate personal efficacy, thoughts, and actions, pursuits, and make adjustments when necessary [3]. Since the agentic perspective (the ability to make things happen intentionally) presupposes individuals, as self-organizing, proactive, self-regulating, and self-reflecting agents, intentionally influence their functioning and life circumstances, the implication is they are both contributors and products of their life circumstances.

When situations arise wherein individuals may be induced to behave inhumanely, they can freely choose not to succumb through self-influence. In essence, moral agency in SCT is exercised through self-sanctions. Moral self-sanctions help ensure people's actions align with their personal moral standards. The overarching implication is the consequences people expect from their behavior regulate their personal conduct, such that "through self-sanctions, people refrain from acting in ways that violate their moral standards and therefore have negative consequences for the self" [4].

In the case of disengagement, however, certain mechanisms need to be triggered or activated to create an environment for social, psychological, and mental maneuvers in which people disengage their moral self-sanctions [3]. This means individuals selectively "turn off" the self-sanctions that ensure their actions conform to moral standards, thus creating an environment for inhumane conduct.

Mechanisms of Moral Disengagement

According to Bandura, there are eight psychosocial mechanisms by which self-censure, sanctions, or control are deactivated selectively, thus enabling the individual to engage in inhumane conduct without negative consequences for the person. Psychosocial mechanisms, selective deactivation, and disengagement of self-sanctions permit certain behaviors by people with the same moral standards. The eight interrelated psychosocial mechanisms consist of moral justification, euphemistic labeling, advantageous comparison, displacement of responsibility, diffusion of responsibility, disregard or distortion of consequences, dehumanization, and attribution of blame [1].

Moral justification involves the cognitive reframing of an unethical function as being in the service of a greater good. People may not engage in unethical or harmful behaviors until they have justified the morality of the action to themselves. The process of moral justification reevaluates what personally and socially is considered harmful and reprehensible by "portraying it as serving socially worthy or moral purposes" [1]. Such cognitive reframing gives people the impetus and moral imperative to preserve their view of themselves as moral agents while inflicting and perpetrating harm unto others. For example, one can find instances of moral justification in military pursuits. People who fight in wars do not change their moral standards or alter their personality when they kill. Instead, they are made to believe and see themselves as fighting ruthless oppressors or dictators, fighting for freedom, protecting cherished values, following religious or ethnic ideology, preserving world peace, or saving humanity from undue subjugation. In essence, moral justification sanitizes and sanctifies the violent means and reframes the morality of killing.

Euphemistic labeling connotes using sanitized language to rename harmful or reprehensible actions to make them appear more benign and less harmful. Its purpose is to make harmful actions responsible while reducing personal responsibility. One way to do this is through sanitizing language even to the extent that killing a human being is no longer morally questionable. For instance, soldiers "waste" people rather than kill them, bombing the enemy is renamed "servicing the target," attacks are seen as "clean surgical strikes," and civilians who lose their lives in a bomb attack are labeled "collateral damage" [1].

The agentless passive voice or style used in describing events creates the impression that harmful acts are the work of nameless forces rather than of people [5]. People present not as real agents of their own acts but rather as if forces move them mechanically. For example, a driver who hit a telephone pole described his actions to the police by saying, "the telephone pole was approaching. I was attempting to swerve out of its way, when it struck my front end" [3]. In euphemistic labeling, inanimate objects sometimes turn into agents in a move to exonerate people and replace words that conjure negative connotations with images or phrases with positive or at least less condemnatory implications.

Advantageous comparison contrasts negative behaviors or actions against even greater wrongdoings or atrocities to make the former seem harmless. It exploits the contrast principle to make reprehensible acts acceptable and righteous. Such exonerating comparison is anchored in moral justification, using utilitarian standards—such as the greatest good for the greatest number of people—and uses the cost–benefit calculus in making ethical judgments. Thus, advantageous comparison deploys this principle by construing nonviolent options as ineffective for achieving desired changes (for the good of all) and presenting adversaries' anticipated threats to show one's reprehensible actions will prevent more human suffering than they cause [1]. For instance, before the United States' invasion of Iraq in 2003, the comparison was between ruthless dictatorships and the threat of weapons of mass destruction. In 2017, the threat posed by North Korea's nuclear capabilities was contrasted with the possibility of a U.S. attack. The whole idea is that an attack will prevent rather than cause more suffering.

The totality of moral justification, euphemistic labeling, and advantageous comparisons account for the most dominant set of psychological mechanisms for disengagement from moral self-sanction. Investing reprehensible conduct and behaviors with high moral purpose "eliminates self-censure, but it engages self-approval in the service of destructive exploits" [3].

Displacement of responsibility occurs when individuals who commit harm consider their actions as emanating from the dictates of authority and are thus free from culpability and self-sanctioning consequences. They feel no personal responsibility for those actions. When people, as moral agents, acknowledge the detrimental effects of wrongdoing, moral control is strong and solid. However, moral self-sanction lessens when a person's responsibility for the injuries caused is reduced, obscured, minimized, or displaced onto others. One instance of self-exemption from gross inhumanities is the Nazi prison commandants who murdered millions of people and claimed they were carrying out orders, thus absolving themselves of personal responsibility.

Diffusion of responsibility is allied closely with displacement of responsibility and aims to minimize the agentic role of action. When diffusing responsibility for detrimental and reprehensible behavior obscures personal agency, moral control is drastically reduced and weakened. Diffusion of responsibility involves dispersing responsibility for one's harmful actions across members of a group [6]. The famous but controversial 1964 case of Kitty Genovese in New York, who was stabbed to death at night in front of her house while about 38 people in her neighborhood watched the incident but did not call the police, is an example of diffusion of responsibility. The research on "Bystander-effect or Bystander-apathy" showed the reluctance of those watching the murder was attributable to the fact they knew others were watching as well. Knowing more people were present helped create the perception of a diffused and divided responsibility [4].

The division of labor can obscure personal agency. It can lead to either collective inaction or collective action. Zimbardo observed that a large group size not only aids in diffusing responsibility but also creates deindividuation when individual group members are easily prone to behave in normally unrestrained ways. Thus, people act more cruelly under group responsibility than when they hold themselves personally responsible for harmful conduct [7].

Distortion of consequences connotes the reduction of the seriousness of the effects of one's harmful acts, thus providing "little reason for the self-censure to be activated" [1]. When people engage in activities that harm others for personal gain or social pressure, their default is to avoid facing the harm they cause or try to minimize it. Moreover, when the effects of one's harmful actions are visible, it is much more difficult to deal with than when they are not known or invisible. For example, modern warfare is culpable for distortion of consequences. People launch bombs, missiles, and drones with computers from remote, safe places such that they do not see or hear the suffering they cause. When moral agents can see and hear the detrimental consequences of their actions, vicariously aroused distress and self-censure serve as self-restrainers [1].

Dehumanization has been described as when something loses all human features, such as feelings, hopes, wishes, and concerns, and instead is seen as an inhuman and subhuman object [8]. The perception of others within the lens of common humanity elicits empathetic emotional reactions through perceived similarity and a sense of social obligation. It is difficult to be cruel to humanized persons without suffering distress from self-censure [1]. However, self-censure for inhumane conduct can be disengaged through dehumanization.

The process of devaluing and dehumanizing victims is an essential component in the perpetration and execution of inhumanities. Dehumanization creates a conducive atmosphere to "mistreat or harm other human beings, ranging from discrimination against them, deprivation of basic rights and opportunities, exploitation to violence, and extreme violence like torture or mass killing" [4]. Therefore, perpetrators of inhumane acts can be engaged in kind acts to people they identify with, while simultaneously meting out cruelty to those they do not identify with.

Haque and Waytz addressed the causes and solutions to dehumanization in medicine. They recognized that dehumanization occurs in hospitals when caregivers and healthcare providers "treat patients less like persons, and more like objects or nonhuman animals" [9]. When dehumanization creeps into the practice of health professionals, it makes them view others "as incapable of fully experiencing joy, pain, and the desire makes it easier to hurt them, without causing feelings of personal distress" [9]. Due to the pain involved in some medical procedures, physicians sometimes feel the need to extricate themselves from their role in committing harm, which is a precursor to empathy reduction. There is the need to minimize the guilt of inflicting pain on patients, even when it is necessary pain that is medically indicated.

In their study on dehumanization within the medical field, Haque and Waytz outlined six possible causes broadly categorized as nonfunctional and functional causes of dehumanization. The first three nonfunctional causes are deindividuating practices (the individual becomes immersed in a group or otherwise anonymized; for instance, physicians who lump patients into stereotypes may be biased in offering them the care they need); impaired patient agency (the perception of patients as impaired in agency due to incapacitation from illness); and dissimilarity (dissimilarity in power between doctor and patient viewed through the lens of superior and subordinate). The other three functional causes include mechanization (thinking of patients as mechanical systems made up of interacting parts for diagnostic and therapeutic purposes); objectification, empathy reduction (failure to consider the patient as a fully social entity that deserves empathy), and moral disengagement (in some painful procedures, physicians extricate themselves from their role in committing harm, which also relates to empathy reduction) [9].

To minimize and fix the evils of dehumanization in medicine, Haque and Waytz suggested the following values be inculcated: individuation (making patients more identifiable and feelings of increased personal responsibility among physicians), agency reorientation (treating patients as agents with the capacity to plan and make choices), promoting similarity (promoting diversity among physicians to match patient demographics), personification and humanizing procedures (highlighting characteristics that distinguish patients from objects or numbers), empathic balance and physician selection (encouraging empathy amidst cognitive objectivity), and moral engagement (decreasing the psychological distance between doctors and patients) [9]. In essence, viewing and treating patients as holistic beings is necessary for physicians to maximize empathy and cognitive problem-solving in every clinical encounter.

Attribution of blame, the last of Bandura's eight interrelated psychosocial mechanisms, is similar to displacement and diffusion of responsibility in that it occurs when a person seeks to blame the victim for bringing suffering on themselves by their disparaging demeanor and belligerent behavior. It is also when a person construes their harmful actions as being triggered by compelling circumstances rather than as a personal decision. As such, shifting the blame on others or compelling circumstances makes retaliation seem self-righteous and excuses the perpetrator's destructive actions.

There is a difference between attribution of blame and displacement of responsibility in terms of who is responsible for the harm. In attribution of blame, victims are made the scapegoats for causing harm to themselves, whereas in displacement of responsibility, the perpetrators shift the blame of their actions to the authorities who gave the orders. In both instances, moral disengagement occurs when the self-exonerating actor blames the victims or the chain of command. For example, there are cases of people being dehumanized based on social, ethnic, religious, or socioeconomic status, such that issues of economic or social injustice are no longer considered; instead, people blame the victims for their situation.

When the eight psychosocial mechanisms are deactivated selectively, it can create an environment for inhumane conduct. For instance, discrimination in daily interaction employs moral disengagement such that "institutionalized discrimination of devalued subgroups in societies takes a heavy toll on its victims. It requires social justification, attribution of blame, dehumanization, impersonalized agencies to carry out the discriminatory practices, and inattention to the injurious effects they cause" [1]. Individuals, in exercising their moral agency, perform harmful actions not through dispassionate abstract reasoning, but through a "self-reactive selfhood" [1]. Therefore, people can show empathy and compassion to their family and friends, while simultaneously being cruel to people they consider outsiders.

The disengagement of self-sanctions from inhumane behavior can focus (a) on conduct, which includes moral justification, euphemistic labeling, and advantageous comparison; (b) on action, which incorporates displacement of responsibility and diffusion of responsibility; (c) the consequences/effects of the action, which involves minimizing, ignoring, or misconstruing the consequences; and (d) on the victim(s) of the action, which includes dehumanization and attribution of blame [4]. When experiencing disengagement, "perpetrators can minimize their role in causing harm by diffusion and displacement of responsibility. It may involve minimizing or distorting the harm that flows from detrimental actions; and the disengagement may include dehumanizing and blaming the victims of the maltreatment" [1].

The issue of moral disengagement is particularly important when considering medical personnel's experiences and interactions with patients and administration. When self-censure, sanctions, or control are selectively deactivated, they can have a devastating impact on patient care.

Dineen examined the moral disengagement of healthcare providers and the effect on the adequate treatment of pain patients experienced. Denying needed resources to control pain does not manifest openly as providers' conscious neglect; instead, it manifests as "subtle, unconscious factors and social-cognitive mechanisms that impact provider decisions" [10]. The treatment of pain is unique because there are no tests, imaging studies, or objective measurements for it. Instead, every assessment depends on the clinical encounter between the physician and the patient. This makes pain treatment prone to bias and to branding patients as "drug-seeking." As such, according to Dineen, healthcare providers who inadequately treat a patient's pain are deploying Bandura's mechanisms of moral disengagement to justify their actions.

Hyatt, in exploring the concept of moral disengagement and its impact on patient safety, stated, "a significant precursor of moral disengagement in healthcare is the moral distress that results from working in an institution in which the dysfunctional systems and processes and/or cultural issues exist related to power differentials or disruptive behaviors" [11]. Moral disengagement among healthcare professionals poses a serious threat to the safety of the patients and the institution's culture and affects the mental health of care providers. Furthermore, besides lower quality of care and diminished autonomy, patients suffer significant and devastating consequences of moral distress and moral disengagement for two reasons: first, when healthcare professionals minimize their communications with patients, patients feel less safe and satisfied with their medical experience, which may hinder their therapeutic progress [12]; second, when healthcare providers estrange themselves emotionally from their patients, their zeal to advocate for the patients' welfare falters [13].

The next chapter explores the concept of ethical climate with particular emphasis on whether and to what extent it plays a role in mitigating the relationship between moral disengagement and moral distress.

References

1. Bandura A. Selective moral disengagement in the exercise of moral agency. J Moral Educ. 2002;31(2):101–19. https://doi.org/10.1080/0305724022014322.
2. Mensch KG. Moral disengagement, hope, and spirituality: Including an empirical exploration of combat veterans [doctoral dissertation]. Exeter: University of Exeter; 2016.
3. Bandura A. Moral disengagement in the perpetration of inhumanities. Pers Soc Psychol Rev. 1999;3(3):193–209.
4. Jackson LE, Sparr JL. Introducing a new scale for the measurement of moral disengagement in peace and conflict research. Con Com Online. 2005a;4(2):1–16.
5. Bolinger D. Language: the loaded weapon. Longman; 1982.
6. Moore C, Detert JR, Trevino LK, Baker VL, Mayer DM. Why employees do bad things: moral disengagement and unethical organizational behavior. Pers Psychol. 2012;65:1–48.
7. Zimbardo P. A situationist perspective on the psychology of evil: understanding how good people are transformed into perpetrators. In: Miller A, editor. The social psychology of good and evil: understanding our capacity for kindness and cruelty. Guilford; 2004.
8. Kelman HC. Violence without moral restraint: reflections on the dehumanization of victims and victimizers. J Soc Issues. 1973;29:25–61.
9. Haque OS, Waytz A. Dehumanization in medicine: causes, solutions, and functions. Perspect Psychol Sci. 2012;7(2):176–86.
10. Dineen K. Moral disengagement of medical providers: another clue to the continued neglect of treatable pain? Houst J Health Law Policy. 2013;13(2):163. https://ssrn.com/abstract=2819461.
11. Hyatt J. Recognizing moral disengagement and its impact on patient safety. J Nurs Regul. 2017;4:15–21.
12. Peleki T, Resmpitha Z, Mavraki A, Manolis L, Rikos N, Rovithis M. Assessment of patients and nurses' opinions on the bidirectional communication during hospitalization: a descriptive study. Health Sci J. 2015;2015(9):1–7.
13. Corley MC. Nurse moral distress: a proposed theory and research agenda. Nurs Ethics. 2002;9(6):636–50.

Chapter 3
The Effects of Ethical Climate on Moral Distress

One question that has to be considered is how much the ethical climate or the organizational culture of a hospital plays a role in determining moral distress and the propensity for moral disengagement among U.S. medical residents. There are various definitions or interpretations of what organizational culture is. For instance, organizational culture has been described as the shared values members of a cooperative group have reflected on, articulated, and accepted as normative [1]. Malloy et al. define it as the "nature of the perception of values, beliefs, and behavior of its members" [2]. When referring to ethical climate as an integral component of organizational culture specifically, Malloy et al. regard it as "the collective perception of what is ethically acceptable within the context of an organization" [2]. Thus, an ethical climate encapsulates an informal yet collective and unanimous perception of what individuals deem acceptable and unacceptable behavior. For Spencer et al., organizational ethical climates incorporate the "shared perceptions of the general and pervasive characteristics of an organization affecting a broad range of decisions" [3]. A positive ethical climate amalgamates an organization's vision with its goals, especially if its values reflect acceptable societal norms consistent with ethical practice. Within the context of health care, Rodney et al. have articulated a moral climate to mean the "implicit and explicit values that drive health care delivery and shape the workplaces in which care is delivered" [4]. McDaniel described an ethical environment as one in which ethical values guide behavior, including setting priorities that provide for the ethical treatment of patients [5].

Within a hospital setting, Olson sees the ethical climate of a hospital as the "organizational conditions and practices that affect the way difficult patient care problems, with ethical implications, are discussed and decided. These conditions and practices are based on the presence of power, trust, inclusion, role flexibility, and inquiry" [6]. Olson asserted they are "those shared perceptions of organizational practices that encompass a wide range of daily administrative, clinical, personal and interpersonal interactions carrying an ethical significance that employees perceive as positive or negative" [6].

A. Ochasi, *The Challenged Resident*, https://doi.org/10.1007/978-3-031-71206-7_3

Numerous studies have been undertaken to ascertain the influence of ethical climate on moral distress. While these studies predominantly have concerned nurses in hospitals, they are worth noting, as the effects of ethical climate on nurse satisfaction, intent to leave, the role of leaders, and so forth are pertinent to medical residents, as interviews with medical residents for my original study have shown. Many of the issues nurses have brought up, from feeling powerless to the perceived lack of ethical behavior on the part of doctors and hospital administrators, correspond to the medical residents' experiences.

When Hart examined the effects of hospital ethical climates on professional and positional turnover intentions of registered nurses, the study concluded hospital ethical climate was the single most important factor in explaining nurses' professional and positional turnover intentions [7]. Rathert and Fleming, in investigating the ethical climate of hospitals in acute care and the moderating role of leaders, found the more benevolent the ethical climate, the more effective the teamwork was among acute care workers [8].

Malloy et al. undertook a broad international study (Canada, Ireland, Australia, and Korea) that explored the perception of 42 nurses on how ethical decisions are made, the hospital role of the nurses, and the extent to which their voices were heard. The study found nurses perceived a "lack of congruence between themselves, physicians, and often patients and their families" [2]. They, furthermore, expressed a sense of powerlessness in the decision-making dynamics and felt vulnerable implementing a care plan for patients for which they had little input. Nurses stated their voices were often silenced, and their approach and understanding of ethical decision-making differed from physicians.

In looking at the various predictors of ethical behavior of nonprofit hospital employees, Deshpande concluded, "ethical behavior of peers, ethical behavior of successful managers, and emotional intelligence have a significant positive impact on ethical behavior of respondents" [9]. The study also found physicians and other hospital employees with political clout within the organization were significantly less ethical than other employees.

Corley et al. added to the understanding of the concept by developing the moral distress scale based on Jameton's theoretical definition of moral distress and Wilkinson's idea of the moral distress model [10]. In a study of 111 critical care nurses in the United States, they found levels of moral distress of moderate intensity occurred with issues of aggressive care, honesty, and action response. For instance, nurses experienced moral distress more frequently when they were required to give a medication intravenously to a patient who had initially refused to take it orally. Of the 111 nurses, 12% had left a nursing position solely due to the effects of moral distress. Corley et al. revised the scale used in the study with a larger sample, which gave rise to the first quantitative measure of moral distress since used and adapted by other healthcare specialties [11]. Corley broadly described moral distress as "psychological disequilibrium, negative feeling state, and suffering experienced when nurses make a moral decision and then either do not or feel that they cannot follow through with the chosen action because of institutional constraints" [12].

Hamric and Blackhall examined the perspectives of nurses and attending physicians on caring for dying patients in the ICU with a particular focus on the links among moral distress, ethical climate, collaboration, and quality of care [13]. The findings revealed both RNs and MDs experience moral distress in the ICU when it comes to futile treatment for dying patients (even though nurses experience it more in such scenarios). The study indicated relatives of patients or the hospital administration often instigated the moral distress both RNs and MDs experienced [13].

In exploring the relationships among ethical climate, ethics stress, and job satisfaction of nurses and social workers in the United States, Ulrich et al. found a "positive ethical climate and job satisfaction protected against respondents' intentions to leave as did perceptions of adequate or extensive institutional support for dealing with ethical issues" [14].

Lutzen et al. investigated the association between work-related moral stress, moral climate, and moral sensitivity among psychiatric nurses in four acute psychiatric wards in Sweden and concluded "moral stress was determined to a degree by the workplace's moral climate as well as by … the mental health staff's moral sensitivity. The nurses' experience of 'moral burden' or 'moral support' increased or decreased their experience of moral stress" [15].

The importance of a hospital's ethical climate cannot be overstated. It is the single most important factor in explaining nurses' turnover intentions. Studies also show a correlation between the intensity of moral distress, ethical work environment, and the frequency of moral distress. In the quantitative study I conducted, interviews with medical residents made it apparent that the same concerns impact medical residents' ability to function effectively in their programs. The ethical climate of a hospital may have a positive or negative influence on the attitudes of medical residents toward their work and, by extension, on how they treat patients.

References

1. Silverman HJ. Organizational ethics in healthcare organizations: proactively managing the ethical climate to ensure organizational integrity. HEC Forum. 2000;12(3):202–15.
2. Malloy DC, Hadjistavropoulos T, McCarthy EF, Evans RJ, Zakus DH, Park I, Lee Y, Williams J. Culture and organizational climate: nurses' insights into their relationship with physicians. Nurs Ethics. 2009;16(6):719–33. https://doi.org/10.1177/0969733009342636.
3. Spencer EM, Mills AE, Rorty MV, Werhane PH. Organization ethics in healthcare. Oxford University Press; 2000.
4. Rodney P, Doane G, Storch J, Varcoe C. Toward a safer moral climate. Can Nurse. 2006;102(8):24–7.
5. McDaniel C. Ethical environment: reports of practicing nurses. Nurs Clin N Am. 1998;33(2):363–72. https://pubmed.ncbi.nlm.nih.gov/9624210/.
6. Olson LL. Hospital nurses' perceptions of the ethical climate of their work setting. J Nurs Scholarsh. 1998;30(4):345–9. https://doi.org/10.1111/j.1547-5069.1998.tb01331.x.
7. Hart SE. Hospital ethical climates and registered nurses' turnover intentions. J Nurs Scholarsh. 2005;37(2):173–7. https://doi.org/10.1111/j.1547-5069.2005.00030.x.

8. Rathert C, Fleming DA. Hospital ethical climate and teamwork in acute care: the moderating role of leaders. Health Care Manag Rev. 2008;33(4):323–31.
9. Deshpande SP. A study of ethical decision making by physicians and nurses in hospitals. J Bus Ethics. 2009;90:387–97.
10. Corley MC, Minick P, Elswick RK, Jacobs M. Nurse moral distress and ethical work environment. Nurs Ethics. 2005;12(4):381–90.
11. Corley MC, Clor T, Elswick RK, Gorman M. Development and evaluation of a moral distress scale. J Adv Nurs. 2001;33(2):250–6.
12. Corley MC. Nurse moral distress: a proposed theory and research agenda. Nurs Ethics. 2002;9(6):636–50.
13. Hamric AB, Blackhall LJ. Nurse-physician perspectives on the care of dying patients in intensive care units: collaboration, moral distress, and ethical climate. Crit Care Med. 2007;35(2):422–9.
14. Ulrich C, O'Donnell P, Taylor C, Farrar A, Danis M, Grady C. Ethical climate, ethics stress, and the job satisfaction of nurses and social workers in the United States. Soc Sci Med. 2007;65(8):708–1719.
15. Lutzen K, Blom T, Ewalds-Kvist B, Winch S. Moral stress, moral climate, and moral sensitivity among psychiatric professionals. Nurs Ethics. 2010;17:213–24.

Chapter 4
Carrying Out the Quantitative Study

As I mentioned in the introduction, the issues I address in this book are based on the findings of a study I conducted with medical residents in the United States that explored the relationship between moral distress and moral disengagement and the moderating role of the ethical climate.

In undertaking the study, two main questions were under consideration—namely, whether to what extent, if any, the frequency and intensity of the experience of moral distress (MD) predicted the propensity for moral disengagement (PMD) among U.S. residents, and whether the perception of the ethical climate (EC) of the hospital moderated the predictive relationship between moral distress and the propensity for moral disengagement among U.S. residents.

Instruments

In the study, I used three instruments to measure one independent variable (moral distress), one dependent variable (moral disengagement), and one moderator variable (ethical climate).

I measured moral distress, the independent variable in this study, using the Moral Distress Scale-Revised (MDS-R) developed by Hamric [1]. I chose this scale for the following three reasons: first, it had the capacity to include more root causes of moral distress; second, it could be used in both ICU and non-ICU settings; and third, it could be utilized appropriately in multiple healthcare disciplines The scale assesses the frequency and intensity of an individual's experience of moral distress. The items are scored by frequency (how often the situation arises), ranging from 0 (never) to 4 (very frequently), and by level of disturbance/intensity (how disturbing the situation is when it occurs), ranging from 0 (none) to 4 (great extent). I obtained the final composite score of moral distress by summing each item's frequency and intensity score, ranging from 0 to 336 [1].

A. Ochasi, *The Challenged Resident*, https://doi.org/10.1007/978-3-031-71206-7_4

The dependent variable in this study was moral disengagement. I measured moral disengagement using the Propensity to Morally Disengage Scale (MDS), designed by Moore et al. [2]. I selected this 16-item scale because of its applicability to a broad sample of adults. In addition, the scale was an appropriate measure that incorporated all the different mechanisms of moral disengagement, rather than only one or a few mechanisms. The tool measured items on a nine-point Likert scale, ranging from "strongly disagree" to "strongly agree," and measured the eight mechanisms activated for moral disengagement as Bandura outlined them: moral justification, euphemistic labeling, advantageous comparison, displacement of responsibility, diffusion of responsibility, disregard or distortion of consequences, dehumanization, and attribution of blame [3].

In addition to the independent and dependent variables, I used a moderator variable to measure the modifying role on the other two variables which, according to Tuckman, can be described as "that factor which is measured, manipulated, or selected by the researcher to discover whether it modifies the relationship of the independent variable to an observed phenomenon" [4]. In the present study, the moderator variable was the ethical climate. I measured it using the ethics environment questionnaire (EEQ) McDaniel developed which offers a measure of ethics in healthcare services. The EEQ is a 20-item questionnaire measured on a five-point Likert scale with response choices ranging from strongly agree (5) to strongly disagree (1) [5]. The items were created following an extensive review of literature in ethics, biomedical ethics, organizational theory, and administrative ethics. To obtain an overall score, I took an average of the summative score with the assigned points on the scale being strongly agree = 5; agree = 4; undecided = 3; disagree = 2; and strongly disagree = 1. The overall mean score of EEQ was 3.1 out of 5.0 and the individual mean scores ranged from 1.8 to 4.8; however, the item raw score was from 1.0 to 5.0.

EEQ provides a good, valid, reliable, and cost-effective measure of ethics in a healthcare organization or setting among multiple practitioners. With its inclusive language and non-site-specific nature, EEQ differentiates the opinions of those practitioners "who thought positively about their work environment from those who thought negatively about it" [5]. In the present study, EEQ specifically measured residents' perception of the ethical climate of their hospitals.

Participants

Given the different specialties in healthcare (e.g., nursing, physical therapy, social work, and so on), this study considered a defined population of medical residents who were currently in their residency programs. A sample of 150 respondents from 14 acute care hospitals in the Eastern and Mid-Western United States received an anonymous web-based questionnaire via email. The residents were from different subspecialties of medicine (such as family medicine, internal medicine, emergency medicine, and critical care) except surgery and pediatrics. Among the questions, residents were asked how long they had been in the residency program so as to ensure they had ample experience with the issue of moral distress. In addition, they were asked about the level of ethics education they had received both in medical school and in their residencies.

Half of the participants in the sample indicated their level of ethics education was low ($n = 48$, or 50%), 32% of participants indicated their level of ethics education was moderate ($n = 31$), while 15% of participants indicated their level of ethics education was high ($n = 14$), and 3% of participants chose "not applicable" ($n = 3$). The highest level of education participants had completed was a professional degree such as MD, DO, or JD ($n = 92$, or 96%). Three participants (3%) had other degrees ($n = 3$) and 1% of participants had a doctoral degree ($n = 1$). Most participants had attended medical school in the United States ($n = 71$, or 74%), 25% of participants attended medical school abroad ($n = 24$), and 1% of participants did not indicate where they attended medical school ($n = 1$).

Table 4.1 presents the demographic frequencies and percentages of the sample. More than half of the participants in the sample indicated they were single and had never married ($n = 53$, or 55%), 44% of participants were married or in domestic partnerships ($n = 42$), and 1% of participants were separated ($n = 1$). The majority of participants identified their ethnicity as Caucasian/White ($n = 53$, or 55%), 21% of participants identified their ethnicity as Asian Pacific Islander ($n = 20$), 6% of participants identified their ethnicity as African American/Black ($n = 6$), and 6% of participants identified their ethnicity as Middle Eastern ($n = 6$). Four participants (4%) declined to identify their ethnicity, 3% of participants identified their ethnicity as multi-racial ($n = 3$), 2% of participants identified their ethnicity as Latino/Hispanic ($n = 2$), and 2% of participants chose "other" ($n = 2$). Finally, most participants were between the ages of 25 and 34 ($n = 71$, or 74%), 23% of participants were between the ages of 35 and 44 ($n = 22$), and 3% of participants were between the ages of 45 and 54 ($n = 3$).

The study collected data through electronic surveys to examine the relationship between moral distress and the propensity for moral disengagement by testing whether the frequency and intensity of moral distress, the independent variable, was predictive of moral disengagement, the dependent variable, among U.S. residents, and the role of the ethical climate, the moderating variable, in moderating the effects of both phenomena. The following two research questions guided the data analyses:

1. To what extent, if any, does the frequency and intensity of [the experience of] moral distress predict the propensity for moral disengagement among U.S. residents?
2. Does the perception of the hospital's ethical climate moderate the predictive relationship between moral distress and the propensity for moral disengagement among U.S. residents?

The first research question addressed the predictive relationship between MD and PMD. The second research question addressed the moderating role of EC.

Table 4.1 Frequencies and percentages for categorical demographic items

Variable	n	%
Are you an intern or resident?		
Intern	21	21.88
Resident	75	78.12
Missing	0	0.00
What is your year of residency?		
Post-graduate year internship (PGY)-1	23	23.96
PGY-2	28	29.17
PGY-3	36	37.50
PGY-4	5	5.21
PGY-5	4	4.17
Missing	0	0.00
What is your specialty in residency?		
Not applicable	2	2.08
Critical care	2	2.08
Dermatology	1	1.04
Emergency medicine	3	3.12
Emergency medicine and family medicine	9	9.38
Emergency medicine and internal medicine	8	8.33
Family medicine	24	25.00
Internal medicine	47	48.96
Missing	0	0.00
What is your gender?		
Female	50	52.08
Male	41	42.71
Missing	5	5.21
How would you rate your level of ethics education from medical school to residency?		
Not applicable	3	3.12
High	14	14.58
Low	48	50.00
Moderate	31	32.29
Missing	0	0.00
What is the highest level of education you have completed?		
Doctoral degree	1	1.04
Other, please specify	3	3.12
Professional degree MD, DO, JD, etc.	92	95.83
Missing	0	0.00

(Continued)

Table 4.1 (continued)

Variable	n	$\%$
Where did you go to medical school?		
Abroad	24	25.00
United States	71	73.96
Missing	1	1.04
What is your marital status?		
Married or domestic partnership	42	43.75
Separated	1	1.04
Single, never married	53	55.21
Missing	0	0.00
Which of the following best describes your race or ethnicity?		
African American black	6	6.25
Asian Pacific Islander	20	20.83
Caucasian White	53	55.21
Latino/Hispanic	2	2.08
Middle Eastern	6	6.25
Multi-racial	3	3.12
Other please specify	2	2.08
Would rather not say	4	4.17
Missing	0	0.00
What is your age?		
25–34 years old	71	73.96
35–44 years old	22	22.92
45–54 years old	3	3.12
Missing	0	0.00

Due to rounding errors, percentages may not equal 100%

Descriptive Statistics

I calculated frequencies and percentages for the categorical demographic questions of the survey. These included items such as residency status, residency year, and the highest level of education. I computed the means and standard deviations for the continuous variable scores, which included MD, EC, PMD, moral distress frequency (MD-F), and moral distress intensity (MD-I).

Frequencies and Percentages

I sent electronic surveys to 150 medical residents and interns from 14 acute care hospitals in the Eastern and Midwestern United States, of which there were 96 complete responses. All specialties in medical residency, except surgery and pediatrics, were eligible to participate. Seventy-eight percent of participants indicated they were residents ($n = 75$) and the other 22% of participants were interns ($n = 21$). The majority of participants (38%, or $n = 36$) were in year PGY-3 of their residency. Twenty-nine percent of participants were in PGY-2 ($n = 28$), 24% of participants were in PGY-1/Interns ($n = 23$), 5% of participants were in PGY-4 ($n = 5$), and 4% of participants were in PGY-5 ($n = 4$).

Almost half of the participants in the sample identified internal medicine as their specialty ($n = 47$, or 49%) and 25% of participants identified family medicine as their specialty ($n = 24$). Nine percent of participants identified emergency medicine and family medicine as their specialty ($n = 9$) and 8% of participants identified emergency medicine and internal medicine as their specialty ($n = 8$). Three participants identified emergency medicine as their specialty and two participants identified critical care as their specialty. Two participants chose "not applicable" ($n = 2$) and 1% of participants identified dermatology as their specialty ($n = 1$). Slightly more than half the participants were female ($n = 50$, or 52%), 43% of respondents were male ($n = 41$), and 5% of respondents did not identify their gender ($n = 5$).

Half of the participants in the sample indicated their level of ethics education was low ($n = 48$, or 50%), 32% of participants indicated their level of ethics education was moderate ($n = 31$), while 15% of participants indicated their level of ethics education was high ($n = 14$), and 3% of participants chose "not applicable" ($n = 3$). The highest level of education participants had completed was a professional degree such as MD, DO, or JD ($n = 92$, or 96%). Three participants (3%) had other degrees ($n = 3$), and 1% of participants had a doctoral degree ($n = 1$). Most participants attended medical school in the United States ($n = 71$, or 74%), 25% of participants attended medical school abroad ($n = 24$), and 1% of participants did not indicate where they attended medical school ($n = 1$).

As indicated in Table 4.1, more than half of the participants in the sample indicated they were single and had never married ($n = 53$, or 55%), 44% of participants were married or in domestic partnerships ($n = 42$), and 1% of participants were separated ($n = 1$). The majority of participants identified their ethnicity as Caucasian/White ($n = 53$, or 55%), 21% of participants identified their ethnicity as Asian Pacific Islander ($n = 20$), 6% of participants identified their ethnicity as African American/Black ($n = 6$), and 6% of participants identified their ethnicity as Middle Eastern ($n = 6$). Four participants (4%) declined to identify their ethnicity, 3% of participants identified their ethnicity as multi-racial ($n = 3$), 2% of participants identified their ethnicity as Latino/Hispanic ($n = 2$), and 2% of participants chose "other" ($n = 2$). Finally, most participants were between the ages of 25 and 34 ($n = 71$, or 74%), 23% of participants were between the ages of 35 and 44 ($n = 22$), and 3% of participants were between the ages of 45 and 54 ($n = 3$).

Table 4.2 Means and standard deviations for MD, MD-F, MD-I, EC, and PMD

Variable	Mean	SD	n
M. distress (MD)	164.86	92.04	51
M. distress-frequency (MD-F)	51.61	24.98	54
M. distress-intensity (MD-I)	59.12	19.08	51
Ethical climate (EC)	3.12	0.48	89
Propensity for M. disengagement (PMD)	3.30	2.03	93

Table 4.3 Results of the reliability analyses for MD, MD-F, MD-I, EC, and PMD

Scale	No. of items	α
M. distress	46	0.96
M. distress-frequency	22	0.97
M. distress-intensity	22	0.94
Propensity for moral disengagement	16	0.99
Ethical climate	26	0.80

Means and Standard Deviations

Table 4.2 presents the means and standard deviations for MD, MD-F, MD-I, EC, and PMD. The average MD score for the sample was 164.86 ($SD = 92.04$). For the MD subscales, the average MD-F score was 51.61 ($SD = 24.98$), and the average MD-I score was 59.12 ($SD = 19.08$). The average EC score was 3.12 ($SD = 0.48$) and the average PMD score was 3.30 ($SD = 2.03$).

Reliability

I used Cronbach's alpha coefficients to conduct a reliability analysis for MD, MD-F, MD-I, EC, and PMD. Table 4.3 presents the results of the reliability analyses for MD, MD-F, MD-I, EC, and PMD. The results indicated all the scales exhibited greater than acceptable reliability, with coefficients in excess of 0.7. Specifically, EC exhibited reliability with a Cronbach's alpha coefficient of 0.80. MD ($α = 0.96$), MD-F ($α = 0.97$), MD-I ($α = 0.94$), and PMD ($α = 0.99$) also exhibited reliability.

Pearson Correlation Analysis

To answer the first research question, I conducted Pearson correlation analyses on the components of MD and PMD, namely MD-F and PMD and MD-I and PMD. I evaluated the correlation coefficients using Cohen's standard, where correlation coefficients from 0.10 to 0.29 indicated a small effect size, those from 0.30 to 0.49

indicated a moderate effect size, and those greater than 0.50 indicated a large effect size [6]. I evaluated the assumption of linearity for each Pearson correlation analysis [7]. Figures 4.1 and 4.2 present the scatterplots of the correlations, which provide a visual interpretation of the relationships between each pair of variables. In both figures, the *y*-axis represents disengagement scores so that higher scores appear toward the upper end of the axis. The *x*-axis represents distress frequency in Fig. 4.1 and distress intensity in Fig. 4.2, such that higher scores are found toward the right

Fig. 4.1 Scatterplot between MD-F and PMD

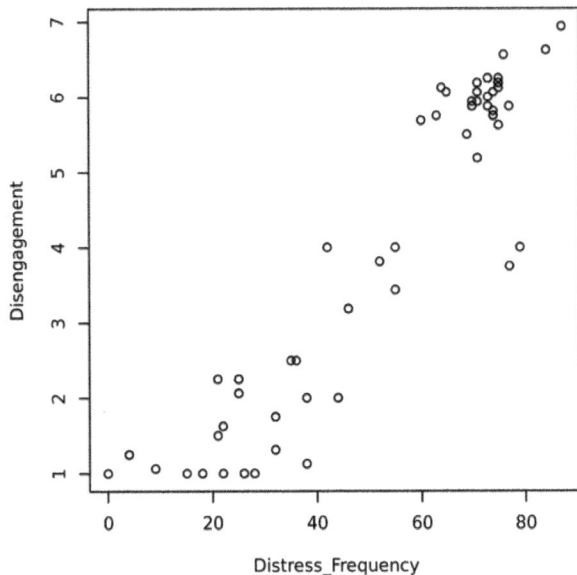

Fig. 4.2 Scatterplot between MD-I and PMD

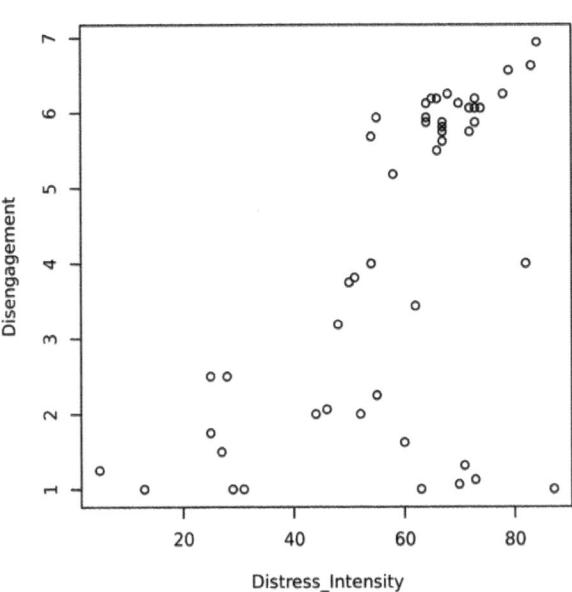

Table 4.4 Pearson correlation matrix between MD-F and PMD

Variable	1	2
M. distress-frequency	–	
PM. disengagement	0.93	–

The critical values are 0.27, 0.35, and 0.44 for significance levels 0.05, 0.01, and 0.001, respectively

Table 4.5 Pearson correlation matrix between MD-I and PMD

Variable	1	2
M. distress-intensity	–	
Propensity for M. disengagement	0.59	–

The critical values are 0.28, 0.36, and 0.45 for significance levels 0.05, 0.01, and 0.001, respectively

end of the axis. Thus, a positive linear relationship would be apparent if data followed a diagonal line beginning near the origin and trending toward the upper right corner of the plot. No curvature is noted in either of the scatterplots; therefore, the assumption of linearity has been met for both analyses.

Tables 4.4 and 4.5 present the results of the Pearson correlation analyses. The findings produced a statistically significant correlation between MD-F and PMD, $p < 0.001$. The correlation coefficient ($r_p = 0.93$) indicated a significant positive relationship between these variables. The findings of the analysis showed that as the MD-F score increased, the PMD score also increased.

In addition, I assessed a statistically significant positive correlation between MD-I and PMD, $p < 0.001$. The correlation coefficient ($r_p = 0.59$) indicated a positive relationship between the variables. The findings of the analysis showed that as the MD-I score increased, the PMD score also increased. These correlational analyses set the stage for linear regression.

Linear Regression Analysis

Question one: to what extent, if any, does the frequency and intensity of [the experience of] moral distress predict the propensity for moral disengagement among U.S. residents?

To answer this research question, I gauged the predictive relationships among MD-F, MD-I, and PMD using multiple linear regression analysis. I conducted this analysis to detect predictive effects from MD-F and MD-I on PMD. Figure 4.3 depicts these effects.

Before conducting the analysis, I weighed assumptions of normality, homoscedasticity, absence of multicollinearity, and lack of outlier. I evaluated normality through a visual examination of a Q–Q, which appears in Fig. 4.4. The Q–Q

Fig. 4.3 Relationship
between MD-F and MD-I
on PMD

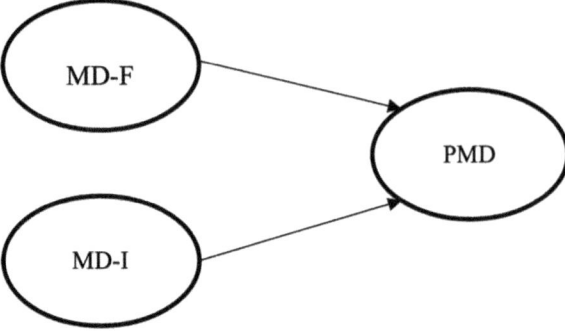

Fig. 4.4 Q–Q scatterplot
testing normality

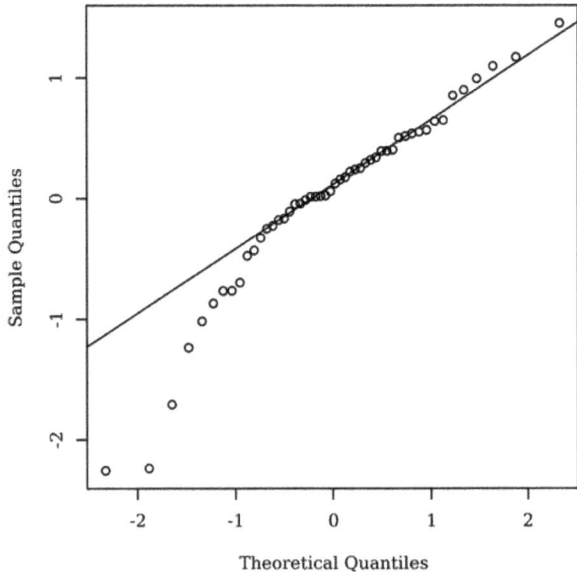

scatterplot displays the data from the regression and shows a perfect normal line for reference when visually assessing the plot. The assumption of normality is met if the data points on the scatterplot follow this perfect normal line. I assessed a mild violation of the assumption of normality because of the slight deviation in the lower tail of the scatterplot, indicating the regression data may not follow a perfectly normal distribution.

I assessed homoscedasticity using a residual scatterplot by plotting the residuals against the predicted values [8], as shown in Fig. 4.5. This plot shows how data are distributed around the regression and can be used to determine whether data are spread consistently around the regression line or have a larger spread at one end of the regression line in comparison to the other. This tendency would be apparent if any funneling was in the plot. Conversely, the assumption of homoscedasticity is met if the data points are distributed randomly about the reference line, as marked

Fig. 4.5 Residuals
scatterplot testing
homoscedasticity

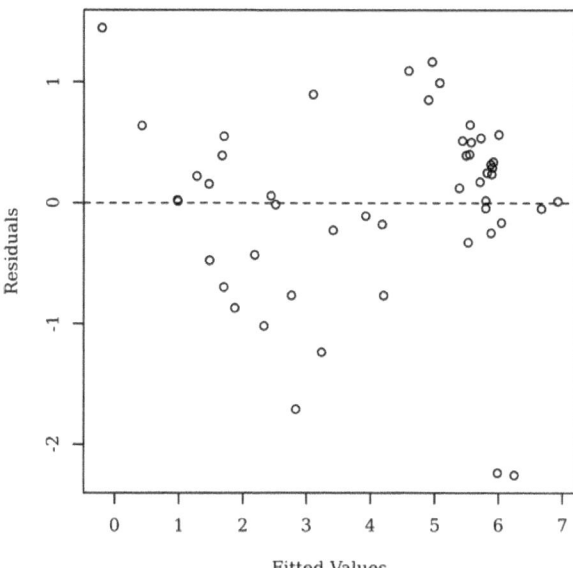

Table 4.6 Variance inflation
factors for MD-F and MD-I

Variable	VIF
M. distress-frequency	1.60
M. distress-intensity	1.60

by the dotted line along the zero value of the y-axis, and there is no curvature in the plot. Based on the lack of funneling or any pattern to the data, the assumption of homoscedasticity was met.

I evaluated the absence of multicollinearity using variance inflation factors (VIFs) to evaluate high correlations between the predictor variables. Table 4.6 presents the VIF values for the predictors. VIFs are a measure of the strength of correlated variables in the regression. Higher values indicate greater correlation and a stronger tendency to invalidate the results due to high multicollinearity. VIF values greater than 10 are considered evidence of multicollinearity [9]. None of the VIF values reached or exceeded 10; therefore, the assumption of multicollinearity was met.

Finally, I evaluated the presence of outliers using studentized residuals. Studentized residuals show how far each datapoint lies from the mean and are measured in units of standard deviation. Based on the degrees of freedom, observations with studentized residuals greater than 3.27 are considered evidence of outliers. To assess these studentized residuals in comparison to the cutoff of 3.27, I plotted these values against the cutoff value and identified them by their observation numbers [10]. Figure 4.6 presents the studentized residuals plot of the observations. None of the studentized residuals were greater than 3.27, indicating a lack of outliers.

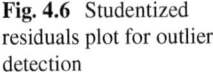

Fig. 4.6 Studentized residuals plot for outlier detection

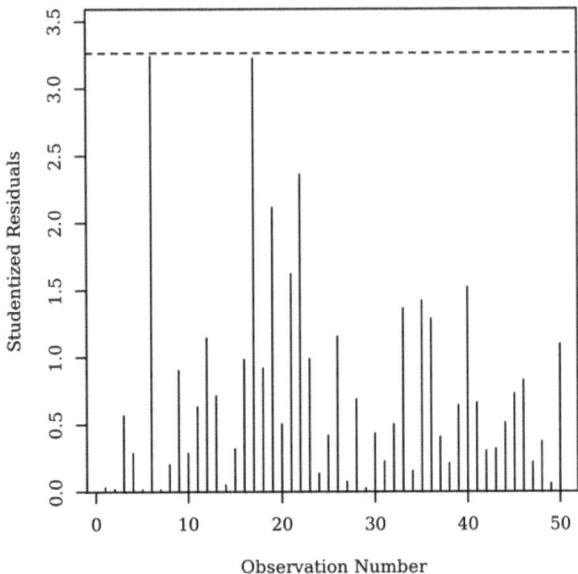

Table 4.7 Results for linear regression with MD-F and MD-I predicting PMD

Variable	B	SE	95% CI	β	t	p
(Intercept)	−0.55	0.37	[−1.29, 0.20]	0.00	−1.47	0.148
M. distress-frequency	0.08	0.01	[0.07, 0.10]	0.91	13.53	<0.001
M. distress-intensity	0.00	0.01	[−0.01, 0.02]	0.03	0.43	0.671

Results: $F(2, 47) = 152.71$, $p < 0.001$, $R^2 = 0.87$. Unstandardized regression equation: PM. disengagement = −0.55 + 0.08 × M. distress-frequency + 0.00 × M. distress-intensity

The multiple linear regression analysis was statistically significant, $F(2, 47) = 152.71$, $p < 0.001$. This finding indicated MD-F and MD-I were related to a statistically significant degree of variation in PMD. The R^2 was 0.87, which indicated MD-F and MD-I accounted for roughly 87% of the variation in PMD. Based on the significant findings for the overall regression, I evaluated the individual values for each predictor. Table 4.7 presents this assessment and the results of the multiple linear regression, with MD-F and MD-I predicting PMD, where contributions of the individual predictors were assessed. MD-I was not a statistically significant predictor of PMD, $B = 0.00$, $t(47) = 0.43$, $p = 0.671$, indicating MD-I did not contribute to the variance in PMD. MD-F was a statistically significant predictor of PMD, $B = 0.08$, $t(47) = 13.53$, $p < 0.001$, indicating MD-F contributed to the variance in PMD. This finding suggested, on average, for every one-unit increase in MD-F, PMD increased by 0.08 units.

Fig. 4.7 Relationship
between MD-F and MD-I
on PMD

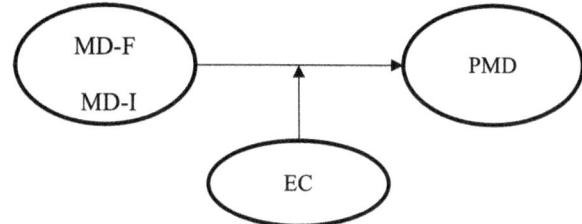

Moderation

Question two: does the perception of the hospital's ethical climate moderate the predictive relationship between moral distress and the propensity for moral disengagement among U.S. residents?

To answer this research question, I conducted a moderation analysis to assess if EC moderated the relationship between MD and PMD. This analysis tested the relationship between the predictor variable MD and the outcome variable PMD and whether the relationship differed based on the PEC value. Thus, the analysis indicated if the relationship between MD and PMD becomes stronger or weaker when EC values are high versus low. This relationship can be seen in Fig. 4.7.

To conduct the analysis, I used mean centering for MD and EC. In the first step, I created a simple effects model using linear regression, with PMD as the outcome variable and MD as the predictor variable. In the second step, I created a noninteraction model by adding EC to the predictor in the linear model in step 1, or the simple effects model. In the third step, I created an interaction model by adding the interaction between MD and EC to the predictors in the linear model in step 2, or the noninteraction model. I conducted assumptions for linear regression analysis for the step 3 interaction model.

Prior to conducting the analysis, I assessed the assumptions of normality of residuals, homoscedasticity of residuals, absence of multicollinearity, and the lack of outliers. In addition, I evaluated normality using a Q–Q scatterplot [8]. The Q–Q scatterplot compares the distribution of the residuals with a normal distribution, which is a theoretical distribution that follows a bell curve. In the Q–Q scatterplot, the solid line represents the theoretical quantiles of a normal distribution. Normality can be assumed if the points form a relatively straight line. Figure 4.8 presents the Q–Q scatterplot for normality.

I evaluated homoscedasticity by plotting the residuals against the predicted values [8]. Figure 4.9 presents a scatterplot of predicted values and model residuals. This plot shows how data are distributed around the regression and can be used to determine whether data are spread consistently around the regression line or have a larger spread at one end of the regression line in comparison to the other. This tendency would be apparent if any funneling appeared in the plot. The assumption of homoscedasticity was met because the points appear randomly distributed with a mean of zero and no apparent curvature.

Fig. 4.8 Q–Q scatterplot
testing normality

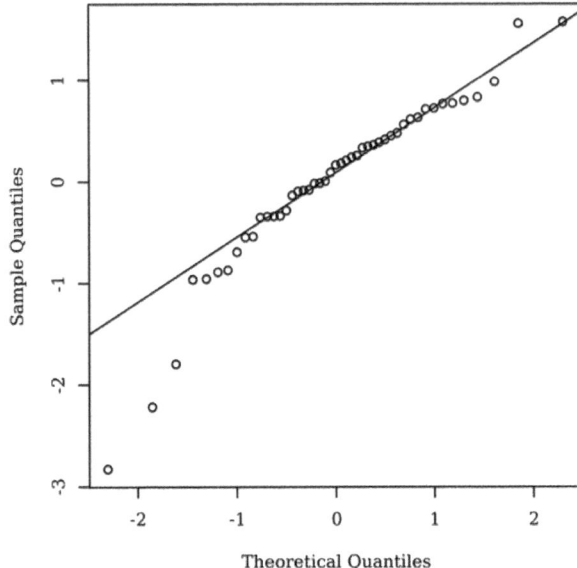

Fig. 4.9 Residuals
scatterplot testing
homoscedasticity

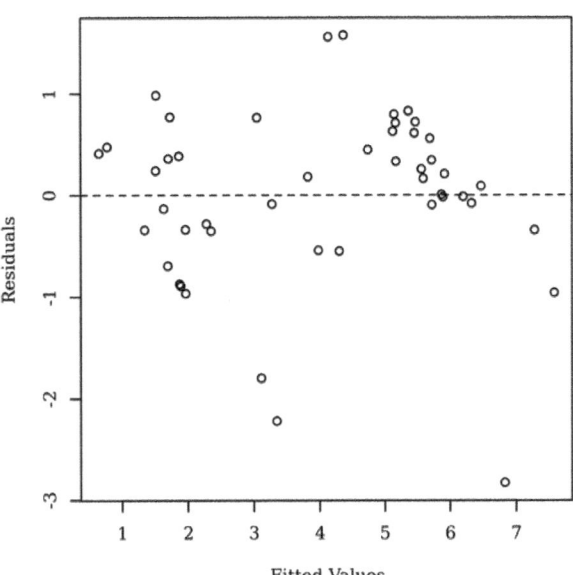

I assessed the absence of multicollinearity using variance inflation factors (VIFs).
Variance inflation factors represent the degree to which correlations between predictors adversely affect the model, where higher values indicate greater correlation
and a stronger tendency to invalidate the results due to high multicollinearity. This
is calculated to detect the presence of multicollinearity between predictors. High
VIFs indicate increased effects of multicollinearity in the model. VIFs greater than

Table 4.8 Variance inflation factors for MD, EC, and MD: ethical climate (EC)

Variable	VIF
M. distress	1.02
Ethical climate (EC)	1.20
M. distress: ethical climate (EC)	1.20

Fig. 4.10 Studentized residuals plot for outlier detection

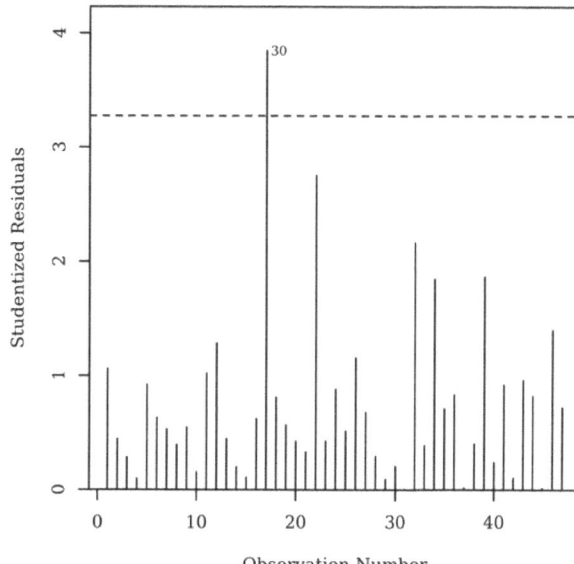

five are cause for concern, whereas VIFs of 10 should be considered the maximum upper limit [9]. All predictors in the regression model have VIFs of less than 10. Table 4.8 presents the VIF for each predictor in the model.

Finally, I evaluated the presence of outliers using studentized residuals. To identify influential points, I calculated studentized residuals, and I plotted the absolute values against the observation numbers [10]. Studentized residuals are calculated by dividing the model residuals by the estimated residual standard deviation, and they show how far each datapoint lies from the mean, as measured in units of standard deviation. As calculated using the degrees of freedom, I considered observations with studentized residuals greater than 3.28 to be evidence of outliers. Figure 4.10 presents the studentized residuals plot of the observations. Observation numbers are specified next to each point with a studentized residual greater than 3.28.

Two conditions must be met for moderation to be supported. First, the causal predictor variable, MD, must significantly predict PMD in the simple effects model from step 1. Second, the interaction model from step 3 must explain significantly more variance of PMD than the noninteraction model from step 2. If either of these conditions fails, moderation is not supported. MD significantly predicted PMD, $B = 0.02$, $t(45) = 15.37$, $p < 0.001$. Therefore, the first condition was met and the second condition was checked. I conducted a partial *F*-test to determine if the interaction model explained more variance in PMD than the noninteraction model. The partial *F*-test, $F(1, 43) = 0.73$, $p = 0.397$, indicated the interaction model did not explain significantly more variance than the noninteraction model. Therefore, the second condition was not met, and moderation was not supported. Table 4.9 presents the results of the simple noninteraction and interaction models. Table 4.10 presents a comparison of the noninteraction and interaction models. To visualize the moderation analysis, I dichotomized EC into high and low categories using a median split. The high category indicates all observations of PEC above the media, and the low category specifies all observations of EC below the median.

Figure 4.11 shows the regression lines for PMD predicted by MD for the high and low categories of EC. This plot shows the strength of the relationship between MD and PMD using two lines. For either of these lines, a steeper slope indicates a stronger relationship, as this would indicate disengagement values (i.e., the *y*-axis) increased more sharply in correspondence to an increase in distress (i.e., the *x*-axis). The black line represents the relationship between MD and PMD for those with a high EC value, while the red line represents the relationship between MD and PMD for those with a low EC value.

Table 4.9 Moderation analysis table with PMD predicted by MD moderated by EC

Predictor	*B*	*SE*	β	*t*	*p*
Step 1: Simple effects model					
(Intercept)	0.47	0.26		1.78	0.081
M. distress	0.02	0.00	0.92	15.37	<0.001
Step 2: Non-interaction model					
(Intercept)	0.41	0.78		0.53	0.597
M. distress	0.02	0.00	0.92	15.07	<0.001
Ethical climate (EC)	0.02	0.24	0.00	0.08	0.940
Step 3: Interaction model					
(Intercept)	4.02	0.13		31.25	<0.001
M. distress	0.02	0.00	0.92	15.05	<0.001
Ethical climate (EC)	0.11	0.26	0.03	0.41	0.685
M. distress: ethical climate (EC)	−0.00	0.00	−0.06	−0.86	0.397

Table 4.10 Linear model comparison table between the noninteraction and interaction model

Model	R^2	*F*	*df*	*p*
Noninteraction	0.84			
Interaction	0.84	0.73	1	0.397

Fig. 4.11 Regression lines for PMD predicted by MD for the high and low categories of EC

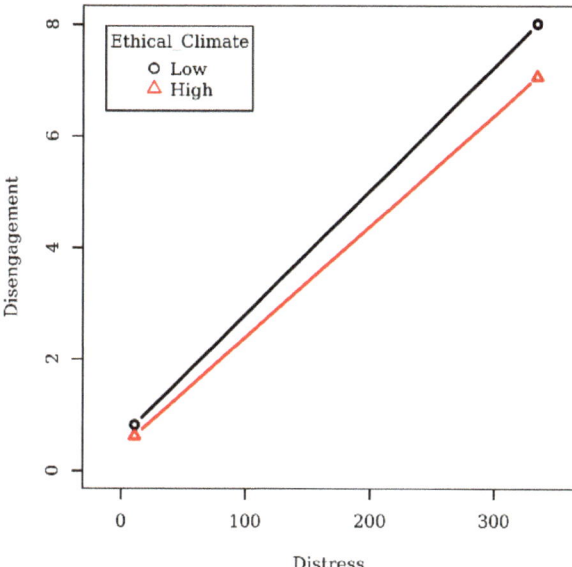

Summary of Quantitative Results

The correlational analysis examined the relationship between the variables: moral distress, the independent variable, and propensity for moral disengagement, the dependent variable. The correlation coefficient (r_p = 0.93) indicated a statistically significant relationship between MD-F and PMD. A statistically significant positive correlation emerged between MD-I and PMD, $p < 0.001$. These results indicated a positive relationship between MD-F and PMD as well as MD-I and PMD, thereby setting the stage for the analysis of RQ1.

The linear regression analysis addressed the first research question: to what extent, if any, does the frequency and intensity of [the experience of] moral distress predict the propensity for moral disengagement among U.S. residents? This was statistically significant, $F(2, 47) = 152.71$, $p < 0.001$. This finding indicated MD-F and MD-I accounted for a statistically significant variation in PMD. The R^2 was 0.87, which indicated MD-F and MD-I accounted for approximately 87% of the variation in PMD. I assessed MD-F and MD-I as individual predictors. MD-I was not a statistically significant predictor of PMD, $B = 0.00$, $t(47) = 0.43$, $p = 0.671$, whereas MD-F was a statistically significant predictor of PMD, $B = 0.08$, $t(47) = 13.53$, $p < 0.001$, indicating MD-F contributed to the variance in PMD. This result partially supports H_1 because MD-F predicted PMD and MD-I did not, if one were to assume the ongoing nature of MD (i.e., frequency) leads to PMD as opposed to intensity.

The moderation analysis for the second research question—does the perception of the hospital's ethical climate moderate the predictive relationship between moral distress and the propensity for moral disengagement among U.S. residents—did not indicate any moderation effect, and I could not reject the null hypothesis. The results showed the perception of ethical climate does not moderate the predictive relationship between MD and PMD.

When interviewing the medical residents for this study, there were certain consistent themes that came up when I asked them to consider whether moral distress predicted moral disengagement and whether the effect of a hospital's ethical climate on the medical residents' experience of moral distress. Chapter 5 discusses their responses and the findings.

References

1. Hamric AB. Empirical research on moral distress: issues, challenges, and opportunities. HEC Forum. 2012;24(1):39–49. https://doi.org/10.1007/s10730-012-9177-x.
2. Moore C, Detert JR, Trevino LK, Baker VL, Mayer DM. Why employees do bad things: moral disengagement and unethical organizational behavior. Person Psychol. 2012;65(1):1–48. https://doi.org/10.1111/j.1744-6570.2011.01237.x.
3. Bandura A. Selective moral disengagement in the exercise of moral agency. J Moral Educ. 2002;31(2):101–19. https://doi.org/10.1080/0305724022014322.
4. Tuckman BW. Analyzing and designing educational research. Harcourt Brace Jovanovich Inc.; 1978.
5. McDaniel C. Development and psychometric properties of the ethics environment questionnaire. Med Care. 1997;35(9):901–14. https://doi.org/10.1097/00005650-199709000-00003.
6. Cohen J. Statistical power analysis for the behavioral sciences. 2nd ed. West Publishing Company; 1988.
7. Conover WJ, Iman RL. Rank transformations as a bridge between parametric and nonparametric statistics. Am Stat. 1981;35(3):124–9. https://doi.org/10.2307/2683975.
8. Bates D, Mächler M, Bolker B, Walker S. Fitting linear mixed-effects models using lme4. J Stat Softw. 2014;67(1):1–48. https://doi.org/10.18637/jss.v067.i01.
9. Menard S. Logistic regression: from introductory to advanced concepts and applications. Sage Publications; 2009.
10. Field A. Discovering statistics using SPSS. Sage Publications; 2009.

Chapter 5
Qualitative Results and Themes

I conducted interviews with experts following the quantitative data analysis of the medical residents' responses. Expert interviews focus on a "person's special knowledge and experiences which result from the actions, responsibilities, obligations of the specific functional status within an organization/institution" [1]. Essentially, expert interviews "serve to establish an initial orientation in a field that is either substantively new or poorly defined, as a way developing a clearer idea of the problem" [2]. The newness and exploratory nature of this project was the primary motivation for using expert interviews to study the correlation between moral distress and the propensity for moral disengagement.

This phase was intended to deepen the conceptual understanding of the three variables in the study and help elaborate the quantitative results. It presented and analyzed interview data in light of the following questions: how does the intensity of the experience of moral distress affect U.S. medical residents; how do the mechanisms deployed by U.S. medical residents to cope with moral distress predict moral disengagement; and how does a hospital's ethical climate influence the experience of moral distress by U.S. medical residents?

The questionnaire consisted of six interview questions (Appendix D) covering the three variables in the study (moral distress, moral disengagement, and ethical climate). The first two questions were about moral distress. I asked the medical residents to describe some incidents they encountered during their residency that caused them moral distress and to articulate their emotions. I also asked them about the frequency and intensity of the distress. The third and fourth questions were about moral disengagement. I asked the residents to describe the coping mechanisms they deployed to deal with moral distress and their feelings about non-compliant patients (whom the residents refer to as "frequent fliers"). The fifth and sixth questions were about ethical climate. Here, I asked the residents to describe the ethical climate of the hospitals they worked in and the level of supervisory/administrative support they received when they experienced moral distress. (For a full view of the Interview Questionnaire, see Appendix A).

© The Author(s), under exclusive license to Springer Nature Switzerland AG 2024
A. Ochasi, *The Challenged Resident*,
https://doi.org/10.1007/978-3-031-71206-7_5

Similar themes and patterns emerged in the residents' responses to all the interview questions. When I asked the residents to describe the incidents that caused them moral distress, five themes emerged:

- Futile and aggressive treatment at the end of life;
- Disregard for the patient's wishes due to pressures from family and inhibiting medical power structures;
- Giving false hope to or deceiving patients;
- Lack of truth-telling and non-disclosure of terminal diagnosis;
- Not doing what is in the patient's best interest due to fear of litigation.

These themes echo Jameton's definition of moral distress as a situation that arises "when one knows the right thing to do, but institutional constraints make it nearly impossible to pursue the right course of action" [3].

Regarding the emotional effects of moral distress on the experts, the following themes emerged:

- Anger due to unsuccessful advocacy for terminal patients;
- Feelings of helplessness and powerlessness;
- Sick, demoralized, and lack of self-worth;
- Sadness, frustration, and anxiety;
- Depression;
- Heartbreak, nightmares, confusion, and mood swings;
- Avoidance and dread of going to work;
- Resurgence of a painful memory.

When it came to coping mechanisms deployed to deal with moral distress, the following themes aligned with moral disengagement:

- Emotional bluntness and indifference;
- Gallows humor;
- Detachment and avoidance;
- Numbness and denial;
- Peer support;
- Strength from faith and prayer.

Similarly, when asked about non-compliant patients who do not follow clinicians' orders, the following themes emerged, reflecting Bandura's mechanisms of moral disengagement [4]:

- Victim blame (attribution of blame);
- Rationalization (moral justification);
- Evading personal responsibility (displacement of responsibility);
- Degradation (dehumanization).

When asked about the ethical climate of the hospitals and supervisory/administrative support with the experience of moral distress, the themes that emerged were:

- Emphasis on law/litigation over ethics;

- Lack of supervisory support for residents;
- Perception of weak and negative ethical climate.

Themes and Responses

There was unanimity among the residents regarding some incidents that caused moral distress though the emotions experienced varied among them. Below are some of the themes that emerged and the effects moral distress had on them.

Futile and Aggressive Treatment for Dying Patients

There was consensus among the residents that aggressive medical treatment perceived to be futile or ineffective for dying patients caused them moral distress. The residents felt that prolonging the dying process was comparable to torture for some patients. One resident spoke about a 49-year-old patient who spent 4 months in the ICU before he died. He was severely malnourished with fluid overload, he developed renal failure requiring hemodialysis, his sternal wound opened to expose his beating heart, and the PEG (percutaneous endoscopic gastrostomy) tube was leaking ascetic fluid:

> Upon the mother's request, aggressive medical treatment continued. This, for me, was sanctioned torture from the mother. Each time I went into that room, I would leave wondering what in the world we were doing to a defenseless human being. This torture continued until the patient died on the 145th day.

Similarly, another resident described the incident, referred to earlier, of the 87-year-old woman with advanced dementia who came to the hospital from a nursing home with an extremely poor prognosis. She was in severe pain, lethargic, and had shortness of breath. Clinicians recommended comfort measures, but the family insisted "everything be done," including a PEG and a tracheostomy:

> They (the family) said something along the lines of "even if she dies on the operating table, that's God's will, or if she dies in an ambulance during transfer, that's her time to go." When family pressures persisted, the GI doctor agreed to put a PEG tube in the dying patient. This [would] have no benefit at all for her. I watched this patient pine away in the ICU for 5 days before she passed away.

Disregard for Patients' Wishes Due to Pressures from Family and Inhibiting Medical Power Structure

In the case of the 95-year-old woman who had broken her hip and had stage four lung cancer with metastasis to the liver and brain, the family insisted on full and aggressive treatment, including surgery, despite the protests from specialists. When the cardiologist was asked why he cleared her for surgery, he replied, "Well, I am helping the family do what they do not want to do, which is making the ultimate decision to transition to comfort measures for their mom." The resident had this to say about her interaction with the attending physician about ignoring the patient's wishes:

> I made my concerns known to the attending who bluntly told me that, in this case, we had to do what the family said and not so much what the incompetent patient said she would have wanted. I felt this woman was unfairly treated by both her family and the care team.

Another resident, who advocated for a patient in a similar dilemma, was told: "'You are a resident, just shut up and do what your attending says.' Such unfortunate cases put you in a corner, and you realize you don't have any power to change the situation for the patient."

Giving False Hope to Patients (Deception)

One resident shared the "unforgettable experience" of a 34-year-old male diagnosed with advanced colon cancer who was given false hope of recovery by the oncologist. He succumbed to the disease after many weeks of aggressive treatment:

> When my attending asked the oncologist about end-of-life/goals of care conversations with the family, he said that such a conversation with a 34-year-old patient would appear as if "we are surrendering and giving up hope." Giving false hopes of recovery to a young patient with an extremely poor prognosis is deceitful. This was an experience I would not easily forget.

Lack of Truth Telling/Nondisclosure of Terminal Illness

Another resident gave an account of how a terminal cancer diagnosis was not disclosed to a 75-year-old woman at the request of her husband:

> I had serious concerns about withholding information from an alert and oriented patient asking about her diagnosis. It bothered me a lot. I also made my feelings known to my attending physician, but he said we should let the family handle it. This was a tormenting few days for my team and the entire staff.

Not Doing What Is in the Best Interest of the Patient for Fear of Litigation

The residents overwhelmingly said they were willing to do what was in the best interest of their patients but could not do so due to threats of litigations from patients' families and proxies. As one resident stated, "The family insisted they wanted the surgery to be done and had threatened to call their lawyer if we failed to do what they wanted." Another said, "I also had another case… where the family threatened the entire hospital with litigation if they removed the ventilator from a teenage son who was brain dead. It was a terrible month for me." Similarly, two other residents noted, "Our legal department strongly requested that we continue to provide aggressive treatment despite the team's concerns that they were futile." And, "At a family meeting a few days later, a copy of the Living Will was presented to the son to reiterate the patient's wishes, but he remained adamant about aggressive treatment and threatened lawsuits."

Effects of Moral Distress on Residents

The frequency and intensity of these distressing experiences produced emotional turmoil among the residents. Many residents mentioned their moral distress was intense and frequently occurred during residency. Two residents had this to say about their experiences, respectively: "I cannot count the number of times I experienced moral distress all these years, but this particular case stood out. I can say that the intensity of that experience was not so great for me." Similarly,

> In terms of the intensity of the experience, nothing comes close to it at all. It was incredibly intense for me. I know moral distress is common and occurs daily in residency, but this one was in a league of its own.

As stated above, certain themes that emerged from the experience of moral distress included anger due to unsuccessful advocacy for terminal patients, feelings of helplessness and powerlessness, and feeling sick, demoralized, and a lack of self-worth. This was compounded by moods of sadness, frustration, anxiety, and depression, which ultimately led to residents experiencing heartbreak, nightmares, confusion, and mood swings. For many, this culminated in avoidance and dread of going to work. The first two themes are reviewed below.

Anger Due to Unsuccessful Advocacy for Terminal Patients

It was clear from the interviews the residents wanted to advocate for patients and do what was right for them. Their inability to do so made them angry. As one resident explained, "I could replay in my head the agony of this patient. I felt as if I did not speak up enough to challenge the decisions of the family, and this made me angry." Two other residents stated, "I was angry at both the family and the GI doc for what they did to the patient. It was even more upsetting that no one even looked at the wishes outlined in her Living Will." And, "I was angry at the mother and the entire team, including the hospital administration, for letting this patient go through this ordeal."

Feelings of Helplessness and Powerlessness

Some of the moral distress the residents experienced stemmed from their feelings of helplessness and powerlessness: "I honestly felt very powerless and helpless at the same time because, as a resident, there is a limit to what you can say or do. No one would even listen if I said anything." One other resident expressed their feelings thus: "I walked out of that conversation feeling helpless because the family who should advocate for the patient was the one causing harm to the patient." Another said,

> Even though I made my concerns known to the attending physician, I felt helpless because the odds were stacked against me. It looked like there was not much I could have done. You know, as residents, the chain of command in every team goes through the attending of records. He seems to have the final say. Disagreeing with an attending physician doesn't look good for you.

Analysis of Moral Disengagement Themes

The frequency and intensity of the distressing experiences led the residents to deploy certain mechanisms to cope with the demands of residency that included emotional bluntness and indifference, gallows humor, and detachment and avoidance, which led to numbness and denial. Some were able to mitigate some of these feelings with the help of peer support and through faith and prayer. I expand on the first three themes below.

Emotional Bluntness and Indifference

Many residents indicated they became emotionally and morally blunt to survive the daily demands of residency. One resident observed,

> I had to convince myself that I could not continue to be this vulnerable to the craziness of dysfunctional families. I built brick walls around my emotions and developed a thick skin. I got into the residency program to graduate and practice medicine; therefore, I needed to protect myself for the future. (Expert 3)

Another noted,

> My professor in medical school once told us that you will be a miserable physician if you ever lose a malpractice lawsuit. This fear has made me tolerate uncomfortable situations and even become indifferent just to graduate from residency without issues. (Expert 2)

Gallows Humor

Some residents used humor to minimize or trivialize the effects of moral distress: "As I said earlier, one way we deal with such situations is to humorize it to minimize its effects on any of us … my colleagues and I laugh about them just to get them off our minds" (Expert 1). Another resident echoed the same sentiments: "Sometimes we make jokes and laugh about some of these experiences just to ensure it doesn't weigh us down. At other times, we try to trivialize the emotions as part of the game" (Expert 7).

Detachment and Avoidance

Some residents used detachment and avoidance as coping mechanisms:

> My natural instinct is withdrawal and avoidance of the unpleasant environment. But being with a team demands that you tag along. However, I wait for the slightest opportunity to withdraw and be alone. This was not a good feeling at all. (Expert 5)

Two other residents observed, "Personally, I have had to call in sick a couple of times to avoid being assigned to patients I felt uncomfortable taking care of" (Expert 1) and "All I do is follow orders from my attending in similar futile situations. It is sad to say that I would walk into a room like a robot these days and leave without showing any emotions" (Expert 3). (See Appendix B.)

Themes That Align with Bandura's Mechanisms of Moral Disengagement

Residents were asked about their perception of noncompliant patients who do not follow clinicians' orders. The following themes reflect Bandura's mechanisms of moral disengagement [4]:

Victim Blaming (Attribution of Blame)

Victim blaming was a recurrent theme for many of the residents. One resident said,

> I had this 20-year-old IV drug user who refused several pleas for rehab and kept coming in and out of the hospital from a drug overdose. It got to a point where I felt no sympathy for him anymore. A couple of months later, he died from an overdose, and his organs were donated. Unfortunately, such patients make their choices and live with the consequences. (Expert 1).

Another observed,

> I've had patients repeatedly come to the hospital for diabetic ketoacidosis by refusing to do simple things like taking insulin. That's irresponsibility. Such patients need to take better control of their health. They can change their destiny by following simple instructions. If they are not accountable, they are responsible for whatever happens to them. (Expert 2)

Expert 5 commented, "To be honest, I feel like smacking them to wake them up. Excuse my language … Such noncompliant patients are fully responsible for whatever happens to their health in the long run. It's hard to sympathize with them, sorry."

Rationalization (Moral Justification)

One resident had to justify the morality of his action for not advocating for patients:

> I got into the residency program to graduate and practice medicine; therefore, I needed to protect myself going forward. If families decide to make irrational decisions for their loved ones, that's their problem. I don't think I should be getting involved. (Expert 3).

Evading Personal Responsibility (Displacement of Responsibility)

Some residents viewed their actions as emanating from the dictates of authority and therefore felt no personal responsibility for those actions: "At other times, we take comfort in the fact that the ultimate decision rests with the attending physician and not us. The attending physician calls the shots, and we go along with the direction he or she wants" (Expert 1). A second resident echoed similar thoughts:

> Even though we worry about prolonging the dying process, there was some solace in the fact that the families' autonomy is the major determinant in such treatments. None of us would want to be named in a lawsuit and normalize such challenging situations to avoid legal trouble. (Expert 2)

Degradation (Dehumanization)

Dehumanization occurs in health care when health professionals treat patients "less like persons and more like objects" [5]. Some residents used language that cast patients as inhumane and subhuman objects. One resident explained,

> One experience that perplexed me was that of a 23-year-old male who overdosed and was recuperating in the ICU. Three days into his recovery, his girlfriend came to visit, and both of them were caught injecting heroin in ICU. We had to call the cops. I guess drug addiction makes people lose their rationality and start acting like animals. This was intolerable for me. (Expert 3)

Analysis of Ethical Climate Themes

The themes that emerged as residents described the hospital's ethical climate centered on their perception that hospitals were concerned with the law and litigation over ethics, that there was a lack of supervisory support for residents, and that there was a weak and negative ethical climate.

Emphasis on Law and Avoiding Litigation over Ethics

Many residents felt there was an undue emphasis on the law over ethics: "Everyone involved in this case felt enormous moral distress. The administration would always defer to the legal and risk department. They were not very supportive. Their immediate concern was avoiding litigation and not so much the distress clinicians were experiencing" (Expert 3). Another resident commented,

> Some of my colleagues, who had issues that got to the risk and legal departments, were told to do everything possible to calm the family to avoid lawsuits. This sent the message that if anything bad happens, you are on your own. (Expert 1)

Lack of Supervisory Support for Residents

Some residents indicated there was a lack of support from supervisors and residency directors:

> I remember when I went to my director to air my views about an attending who was constantly demeaning residents. What I heard from him shocked me. He told me: "You are here to complete your residency and not get into fights with the attending." He also said that attending physicians were like gods when he did his residency years ago, and residents dare not challenge them. After this sad encounter, I decided not to go to him again for any support. (Expert 2)

Perceptions of a Weak and Negative Ethical Climate

The residents overwhelmingly described the ethical climate of their hospitals as being negative:

> I'm not even sure if there was any ethics recourse for people who've had similar experiences. I felt abandoned. I heard from some of my colleagues that there was an ethics committee, but I do not know how they operate or when they meet. I would simply describe the ethical culture as lax. Everyone does what he or she believes is right as long as they stay under the radar. (Expert 4)

(See Appendix C).

References

1. Littig B. Interviews, expert. In: Badie B, Berg-Schlosser D, Morlino L, editors. The international encyclopedia of political science. Sage; 2011.
2. Bogner A, Menz W. The theory-generating expert interview: epistemological interest, forms of knowledge, interaction. In: Bogner A, Littig B, Menz W, editors. Interview experts. Palgrave Macmillan; 2009.
3. Jameton A. Nursing practice: the ethical issue. Prentice-Hall; 1984.
4. Bandura A. Moral disengagement in the perpetration of inhumanities. Pers Soc Psychol Rev. 1999;3(3):193–209.
5. Haque OS, Waytz A. Dehumanization in medicine: causes, solutions, and functions. Pers Psychol Sci. 2012;7(2):176–86.

Chapter 6
Discussion of Findings

In the quantitative phase of the study, I examined the relationship between moral distress and the propensity for moral disengagement by testing whether the frequency and intensity of moral distress, the independent variable, is predictive of moral disengagement, the dependent variable, among U.S. residents, and the role of the ethical climate, the moderating variable, in moderating the effects of both phenomena. A preliminary correlational analysis revealed a statistically significant relationship between the frequency of moral distress and the propensity for moral disengagement. Similarly, the findings indicated a statistically significant positive correlation between the intensity of moral distress and the propensity for moral disengagement among U.S. residents.

I designed the first research question to examine whether the frequency and intensity of moral distress predicted the propensity for moral disengagement among U.S. residents. The analysis found this relationship to be statistically significant. However, when I assessed moral distress frequency and moral distress intensity as individual predictors of moral disengagement, moral distress frequency was a higher statistically significant predictor of moral disengagement than moral distress intensity. When combined, both moral distress frequency and moral distress intensity were found to be significant predictors of moral disengagement, but as individual predictors, moral distress frequency predicted moral disengagement more than moral distress intensity.

The second research question explored whether the perception of the hospital's ethical climate moderated the predictive relationship between moral distress and the propensity for moral disengagement. The study found perception of the ethical climate does not moderate the predictive relationship between moral distress and the propensity for moral disengagement.

The fact that the ethical climate did not moderate the predictive relationship between moral distress and the propensity for moral disengagement could have many explanations. One possible reason why the moderation analysis was not supported in this study could be the insular culture of residency itself that shields

© The Author(s), under exclusive license to Springer Nature
Switzerland AG 2024
A. Ochasi, *The Challenged Resident*,
https://doi.org/10.1007/978-3-031-71206-7_6

residents from the influence of external factors, such as the ethical climate of the hospital. Residency training has a unique culture that isolates residents from the broader culture of the hospital. Unwritten codes and ethos insulate residency programs, sometimes precluding the broader organizational climate from permeating through [1]. Broadly, there is a difference in the mindset of a regular health care employee, such as a doctor, nurse, or social worker, who wants to work and engage with the organization for years and a resident who sees the organization as a temporary place of training before moving on to find employment elsewhere. This difference may affect how each group interacts with the organizational culture and conforms to the ethical norms. In other words, residents may have a transient outlook on what happens around them, as opposed to regular employees who may take a more long-term perspective on events around them.

The temporary and transitory mindset could predispose residents to condition themselves to conform to the culture of residency, as opposed to the hospital culture, to survive the training program. This form of conditioning might make the ethical climate of the hospital unable to impact the mindset of residents. Systematically, a strong hierarchical structure characterizes the culture of residency. From the beginning of medical schools, doctors have been socialized to respect hierarchy and not challenge authority [2]. The medical hierarchy conditions residents to accept their position at the bottom of the power structure. They are expected to endure harsh treatments and distressing situations without complaint. There is an expectation they need to prove themselves worthy of the profession [3]. Consequently, morally distressing situations are likely not addressed due to these unwritten rules governing residency [1]. This explanation is compatible with Hilliard et al.'s study that identified the lower status of residents in the hierarchy of medical care teams as a source of moral distress, especially when there is a disagreement between those residents and the senior staff [4].

Other unique components of the residency culture that differ from the larger hospital culture are "anger and fear, intimidation and humiliation, alienation and disillusion" [1]. Residents believe their career progression is dependent on attending physicians, consultants, and faculty because these superiors might write reference letters for future employment. Residents might feel as if they need to stay on good terms with these superiors, irrespective of their personal feelings about their behavior. As such, residents might not challenge forms of humiliation and dehumanization for fear of angering superiors. Garelick and Fagin noted that for some residents the "differences in power and status, and dependence on references, places juniors in invidious positions when they experience problems in their relationships with trainers" [5]. Thus, the sense of futility in challenging or seeking redress when problems arise may lead to alienation, disillusionment, numbness, and detachment [1, 3]. This power imbalance may be present in the larger hospital climate, but it pales compared to the residency world. The unique and insular structure of residency is one possible explanation why the larger hospital's ethical climate may not affect residents. The explanation above somehow aligns with the findings by Dzeng et al. who noted that in light of perceived helplessness during residency, "physician trainees can become emotionally detached and cynical, and may dehumanize their patients in order to protect themselves" [6]. Residents' instinct to survive the training may trigger coping mechanisms such that the ethical climate of the hospitals may not have any effect on the individual residents. According to Hilliard et al., powerlessness and helplessness inherent in the structure of residency may explain why residents who experience moral distress feel they do not have open, safe, and necessary supervisory support to discuss their concerns, which may lead residents to create coping mechanisms out of the sense of the futility of challenging the system [4].

A Summary of the Qualitative Portion of the Study

I undertook the qualitative phase of the study to explain or elaborate the quantitative results. To do so, residents' interpretation of their experiences of moral distress and the meaning (or feelings) they ascribed to these experiences were sought out. Three research questions guided the experts' recollection of moral distress, moral disengagement, and ethical climate. The residents described the incidents that caused them moral distress as frequent and intense. Some of the themes that emerged were futile and aggressive treatment at the end of life; disregard for patient's wishes due to pressures from family and inhibiting medical power structure; giving false hope to or deceiving patients; lack of truth-telling, nondisclosure of terminal diagnosis; and not doing what is in the patient's best interest due to fear of litigation.

The residents described their feelings (emotions) induced by moral distress. Some feelings or emotions they identified were anger, helplessness, powerlessness, demoralization, lack of self-worth, sadness, frustration, anxiety, and depression. These moral distress themes corroborate the results of the quantitative section of the present study that showed high levels of moral distress among U.S. residents.

The residents also identified emotional bluntness, indifference, gallows humor, detachment, avoidance, numbness, and denial as some of the coping mechanisms deployed to deal with moral distress. One described developing a "'thick skin' to withstand any morally challenging situation," while another admitted to becoming "indifferent just to graduate from residency without issues." In addition, when I asked residents about noncompliant patients who do not follow clinicians' orders, the concepts and themes that emerged reflected four of Bandura's mechanisms of moral disengagement: (a) victim blaming (attribution of blame); (b) rationalization (moral justification); (c) evading personal responsibility (displacement of responsibility); and (d) degradation (dehumanization). These results are similar to the findings of the quantitative phase, which showed a correlation between moral distress and moral disengagement [7].

The residents' assessments of their hospital's ethical climate on the whole were negative. They expressed a lack of supervisory and administrative support whenever they dealt with morally distressing situations. As one resident expressed, "My hospital has an ethics committee that meets once every 2 months. Other than that, I think most people decide what is ethical for them. The unwritten rule is not to get caught." Another resident contributed, "I would describe the ethical culture as lax. Everyone does what they believe is right as long as you stay under the radar."

The administration was more concerned with avoiding litigation than addressing the moral concerns of the individual residents. The residents felt the negative ethical climate might have amplified their experience of moral distress. This result did not corroborate the findings of the present study's quantitative phase, even though the quantitative phase examined whether the ethical climate moderated the relationship between moral distress and moral disengagement. Granted that the qualitative and quantitative approaches were different, some of the themes that emerged in the qualitative phase seemed to support the unproven hypothesis of the qualitative phase, which theorized that a strong or positive ethical climate would ameliorate the predictive relationship between moral distress and moral disengagement.

In summary, the two phases of this research supported the claim that when moral distress frequently occurs with high intensity among U.S. medical residents it increases their propensity to disengage morally. Furthermore, the ethical climate plays a vital role in the residents' experience of moral distress.

Implication for Leadership of Residency Programs

As the study demonstrated, the frequency and intensity of moral distress make medical residents susceptible to moral disengagement, which ultimately affects patient care. The residents' perception of the ethical climate also affects how they experience moral distress. Thus, the challenge for the administration and leadership of healthcare institutions, especially residency directors, is recognizing the problem this phenomenon poses to residents and putting mechanisms in place to address it whenever it occurs. This is necessary to break the cycle of indifference that has dogged the issue of moral distress in residency programs. Unaddressed moral distress not only affects the residents and the care they provide to patients but also perpetuates the culture of inaction and denial of a critical issue in the medical establishment. Berger described the severe impact of unaddressed moral distress thusly: "Morally blunted residents who become morally blunted attending physicians may disproportionately engage in negative mentoring, thereby exacerbating and perpetuating this problem" [8].

Generally, there is a need to change the culture of stoicism that is endemic in the medical community. There is an unchallenged belief that medicine is a demanding profession and only tough people survive the rigors of medical training. Consequently, an admission of any feelings of distress during medical training is perceived as a sign of weakness. In order to break through this superannuated concept of stoicism within the medical profession, leaders, hospital administrators, and residency directors should openly recognize and discuss the reality of moral distress in residency, as is evident in medical literature and the findings of this study. Such moves would elevate the awareness of this phenomenon as a problem in need of solutions. It would be difficult to initiate and sustain a cultural change in the medical community about moral distress without the creative direction and commitment of those in leadership. Nor would it require any structural readjustments to effect this change. A good start would be leaders recognizing and prioritizing the threat that moral distress poses to residents and patients' emotional and physical well-being, just as many in the medical community are currently grappling with the issue of physician burnout.

In line with the need to counteract the medical culture of stoicism, the Association of American Medical Colleges (AAMC), which oversees all 152 accredited U.S. and 17 accredited Canadian medical schools, should require a more robust ethics curriculum to be integrated into training and clinical rotations of third- and fourth-year medical students. Emphasis should be placed on situations that negatively impact the physical and emotional health of prospective physicians, such as moral distress, burnout, and stress. Similarly, the Accreditation Council for Graduate Medical Education (ACGME), responsible for the accreditation of residency programs, already requires hospitals and medical centers to have ethics curricula and a mechanism for residents to freely discuss ethically and emotionally challenging experiences they encounter during residency. However, given the importance of the emotional health of residents to both themselves and their patients, there is a need to intensify efforts at the national level to address issues of moral distress.

The following mechanisms should be implemented at the hospital level to create awareness and promote an ethical environment that welcomes and encourages discussions of morally challenging experiences. First, the Joint Commission on the Accreditation of Healthcare Organizations (JCAHO) passed a mandate in 1992 that all JCAHO-approved hospitals must put some mechanism for discerning and addressing ethical concerns [9]. The reality is some hospitals have functional ethics committees, while others exist only on paper. In light of the present study's findings, every hospital with a residency program should have an active ethics committee or revive one that has become moribund; general ethics committees should create a subcommittee or team tasked with helping residents discuss their experiences of moral distress in a safe and supportive manner; the team should be interdisciplinary and should consider including at least one subject matter expert on moral distress. Such a team would make the residents comfortable discussing their feelings in a smaller setting instead of a full ethics committee, which residents might find overwhelming or intimidating.

While a committee might not encapsulate fully an entire hospital's climate, addressing the moral distress of residents is a small, albeit necessary, component of the solution. This recommendation may be fraught with problems given the misperceptions of ethics committees at different institutions. One common misperception is ethics committees are extensions of the hospital administration and may not act as the neutral arbiters they were designed to be. Some people also believe ethics committees are rubber stamps for physicians when they disagree with patients and their families, especially given that most chairs or co-chairs of the committees are physicians. While the neutrality and objectivity of ethics committees are legitimate concerns, there is a shortage of neutral structures in hospitals to handle issues of moral distress when they arise. Despite the encumbrances of ethics committees, they still have the makeup to be unbiased judges. In this situation, the perfect should not be the enemy of the good. Hospitals can start with this sub-team of the committee and reevaluate or tweak the structure over time to address the moral distress of residents.

Some hospitals may have situations where the ethics committee is either nonexistent or dysfunctional. A viable alternative would be to create a confidential support group (CSG) that offers residents a confidential forum to discuss sensitive and morally distressing experiences that they may not feel comfortable discussing with their immediate supervisors or human resources. The hospital's administration, residency faculty, and ACGME would appoint members of this group based on knowledge and expertise in addressing residents' moral distress and wellness. The CSG should be neutral so residents can feel free to contact any group member anytime to discuss issues. The issues discussed would be kept strictly confidential within the support group and members of the group would help provide reasonable services to assist the residents in their distress.

Furthermore, hospitals should institute ethics programs such as grand rounds, didactic sessions, and weekly teaching rounds with an emphasis on the emotional health of residents. Residency directors, faculty, and attending physicians who mentor residents should be encouraged to participate in these programs. Including mentors in these programs is essential to reorient them about the reality and impact of moral distress. As Berger noted, "Unfortunately, most physician mentors had poor support for their own moral distress during their training experiences … and may not fully appreciate its impact or even validate its existence" [8]. All stakeholders in the medical power structure need to recognize and embrace this phenomenon and do all they can to support residents who experience distress. The shared and collective responsibility of all stakeholders can create awareness of this issue plaguing residency programs.

The unexpected emergence of COVID-19 had a direct impact on medical personnel who were unprepared for the scope of the illness and the number of patients who were suddenly under their care. In the case of medical residents, many not only felt unprepared for the responsibilities they faced, but were also worried about the impact on their training and education. In the next chapter, I examine in more detail how the impact of coping with COVID-19 led many residents to experience moral distress and burnout.

References

1. Crowe S, Clarke N, Brugha R. 'You do not cross them': hierarchy and emotion in doctors' narratives of power relations in specialist training. Soc Sci Med. 2017;186:70–7.
2. Lempp H, Seale C. The hidden curriculum in undergraduate medical education: qualitative study of medical students' perceptions of teaching. Br Med J. 2004;324(7469):770–3.
3. Mistry M, Latoo J. Bullying: a growing workplace menace. Br J Med Pract. 2009;2(1):22–6.
4. Hilliard RI, Harrison C, Madden S. Ethical conflicts and moral distress experienced by paediatric residents during their training. Paediatr Child Health. 2007;12(1):29–35.

5. Garelick A, Fagin L. Doctor to doctor: getting on with colleagues. Adv Psychiatr Treat. 2004;10:225–32.
6. Dzeng E, Colaianni A, Roland M, Levine D, Kelly MP, Barclay S, Smith TJ. Moral distress among American physician trainees regarding futile treatments at the end of life: a qualitative study. J Gen Intern Med. 2006;31(1):93–9.
7. Bandura A. Selective moral disengagement in the exercise of moral agency. J Moral Educ. 2002;31(2):101–19.
8. Berger JT. Moral distress in medical education and training. J Gen Intern Med. 2013;29(2):395–8.
9. Annas G, Grodin M. Hospital ethics committees, consultants, and courts. AMA J Ethics. 2016;18(5):554–9. Published 2016 May 1. https://doi.org/10.1001/journalofethics.2016.18.5.sect1-1605.

Chapter 7
Residency During COVID-19

This study was completed at the beginning of the COVID-19 pandemic. The onset of COVID-19 had a profound effect on the nation as millions died from the virus, lockdowns were implemented, and unemployment skyrocketed, among other dramatic changes within our society. The virus's effect on the medical field was equally overwhelming. Within the hospital setting, healthcare providers faced having to implement crisis standards of care, shortages, and rationing of supplies, and long working hours. The burdens on healthcare workers, many of whom were unprepared for the obligations suddenly placed on them, led many to experience moral distress and burnout. Medical residents were impacted directly in several ways, from their education and training to the fear they themselves would contract COVID-19 and spread it to loved ones. This chapter documents factors that contributed to healthcare workers' and medical residents' moral distress and burnout when working under the conditions COVID-19 presented.

Education

In describing the impact of the pandemic on residency training, Jaqua explains how the pandemic not only affected the way residents took care of patients but also the residents' education. As she describes,

> [COVID-19] led to many modifications for safety reasons within the clinics and hospitals that resulted in decreased volumes of procedures, face-to-face teaching, hands-on training, and skill-based activities. Elective rotations had to be cancelled, reducing interpersonal connections in favor of social distancing and home isolation. The residents' clinical skills competence in doing a physical exam weakened as they no longer [had] access to patients under supervision. The conventional bedside teaching where residents and faculty can ask patients questions in real-time and have essential discussions as a team had to be discontinued [1].

© The Author(s), under exclusive license to Springer Nature Switzerland AG 2024
A. Ochasi, *The Challenged Resident*,
https://doi.org/10.1007/978-3-031-71206-7_7

Laloo et al., too, reported the pandemic had the effect of impeding medical training and learning through restrictions that were imposed, including a decline in face-to-face lectures, tutorials, ward-based teaching, simulation sessions, and morbidity and mortality meetings [2]. In order to make sure students kept up with their medical training, hospitals utilized online platforms. This included weekly lectures for residents and grand rounds sessions. In some instances, instructors cancelled classes altogether, as the physicians who taught them were not prepared to present them online [3]. Another impact of COVID-19 on medical education was the cancelling of medical conferences. These conferences and the associated presentations that medical students give are essential to building up medical students' resumes and applications for residency. As Ferrel and Ryan observed, regarding the cancellation of medical conferences,

> Many medical students … also lost the opportunity for personal development through conference presentations. These presentations play a large role in distinguishing applicants during the residency application process, and therefore these lost opportunities have the potential to be a serious detriment to medical students' career trajectory [4].

Long Working Hours

The number of patients admitted to hospitals and the lack of healthcare workers meant residents were forced to work shifts they were psychologically unprepared for. As Anna Yap, MD—at the time, a second-year resident in the UCLA-Ronald Reagan/Olive View emergency medicine program—explained,

> These shifts are harder than I cerebrally thought they would be … Having to wear personal protective equipment [PPE] all the time is uncomfortable. The worry about, "Am I going to get sick? Am I putting this on correctly? What if I do something wrong?" There are so many what-ifs and it compounds anxiety, along with increased patient anxiety as well [3].

Jaqua further remarked that hospital shifts were exhausting, "not only because of the long hours and multiple days working in a row but also the constant fear of spreading the virus to a loved one" [1].

Safety Protocols

Needing to adhere to extreme safety protocols added to residents' stress. Not only was the personal protective equipment (PPE) extremely uncomfortable, but some also felt the need to dress in full PPE meant that they were giving their patients substandard care, as they had to take time to ensure they were protected fully, especially in cases of emergencies [5]. In a study looking at factors that distressed registered nurses, one of them was that "providing care while wearing burdensome PPE changed health care delivery, diminishing interactions with patients and compromising communication due to masks and shields" [6].

Fear of Getting the Virus

Norman et al. reiterated that front-line workers were constantly concerned they would get the virus [7]. As many residents stated, their fear was not only for themselves but also for their loved ones and other patients they tended to. In a study by Messner et al. one resident remarked,

> You know, the emotional toll was fairly difficult because, you know, that there's a lot of at first anger and then frustration and then fear about potentially getting ill, and then finding out being one of the essential workers that I would ultimately be returning to work and potentially be exposed to what learning is to be a deadly pandemic type of a virus [8].

Compromising Their Integrity

Jacobs and Manfredi pointed out that during the height of the pandemic, clinicians felt they were constantly compromising their integrity, as they had to negotiate between what they could do and what they wanted to do as a result of resource shortages [9]. According to Jacobs and Manfredi, moral distress occurred among nurses working in critical care settings when they faced

- Having to continue artificial life support despite the perception of futility;
- Inadequate communication about end-of-life care between clinicians, patients, and families;
- Perceived inappropriate use of healthcare resources;
- Inadequate staffing or staff … trained to provide the required care;
- Insufficient pain relief for patients;
- Unclear communication with patients and families, resulting in "false hope" [9].

Jacobs and Manfredi further emphasized residents were at risk for moral distress because, while they had the responsibility of implementing care they had no authority to design the plans [9]. What they were feeling, in fact, was the very issue I addressed in Chap. 1: feeling powerless in the fact of being, as Dzeng et al. put it, "subordinate but on the front line" [10].

Rationing of Equipment

Another problem many faced at the beginning of the pandemic was the anticipated shortage of equipment needed for patients with Covid-19. That meant having to make choices concerning who was to receive what care. In the early days of the pandemic, one doctor warned, that the effect of making such decisions would have an adverse effect on those who had make those judgements: "The angst that clinicians may experience when asked to withdraw ventilators for reasons not related to the welfare of their patients should not be underestimated … . It may lead to debilitating and disabling distress" [11]. While COVID-19 progressed and rationing supplies became a reality, many healthcare workers were both distressed and outraged by the conditions they had to work in. As one clinician exclaimed, "I took an oath to care for and protect my patients. How could I possibly tell my patients we have no more ventilators to put them on?" while another stated, "I'm risking my life caring for patients on the front lines, and it's unacceptable that I'm not even being provided with adequate PPE!" [12]. For many healthcare workers, constantly needing to make assessments and often take actions against their deeply held beliefs led to profound feelings of moral distress.

Changing Policy Factors

An issue that was often a stressor during the pandemic were the effects of policy factors, as nurses pointed out in interviews in a study Sims et al. undertook. In response to the continuous changes in procedures, one nurse commented,

> Literally from a day-to-day basis, you can show up, and things are being done different than they were the day before when you were there. From shift-to-shift, you're getting different information. Then now also, every day you're being blasted with new information, long memos about new procedures about things [13].

All of these elements contributed to moral distress in residents, as well as healthcare workers in general, and were predictors of burnout, depression, anxiety, and PTSD.

Telehealth

The transition to telehealth as a way to keep in contact with patients was an added stressor for residents and professionals. Many healthcare workers had inadequate equipment. Often, elderly patients, in particular, were not familiar with or had little knowledge of the technology, which resulted in scheduled time slots being taken up with coaching the patients on how to get online or how to navigate the programs leading to "feelings of confusion and lack of control" on the part of healthcare workers [14]. Messner et al. wrote that one resident stated,

> I think there was definitely a learning curve at the beginning, trying to figure out how to do a physical exam and assessment over the phone. I think that there were a few times when I felt limited in my ability to diagnose something accurately and still able to listen if there's any red flags that need urgent or emergent evaluation [8].

Feelings of Isolation

Social isolation was another stressor that impacted medical students during COVID-19. Patterson et al. described how medical students were affected:

> Students woefully watched ill patients suffer alone because family members were prohibited from visiting due to hospital restrictions. This painful disconnection from patients was exacerbated by the students having to wear masks that hid their facial expressions, making them feel even more incapable of comforting their sick patients [14].

Evolution and Response to Moral Distress

In studying how COVID-19 led to moral distress among health workers, Daubman et al. noted a pattern that evolved, which they described as the evolution and response to moral distress [12]. The first was indignation, where "the clinician is shocked and horrified by the conditions encountered, the severity of suffering, and a lack of resources" [12]. The second was resignation, where "clinicians go through the motions and continue to care for patients but feel disillusioned" [12]. Finally, there is the acclimation stage, where "a productive rhythm develops as teams coalesce and are galvanized by a shared sense of purpose" [12].

Daubman et al. stated the importance of this framework was to recognize and provide guidance for those who were in distress. Being able to recognize the pattern many health care workers experienced could help them recognize that what they were feeling was common among their colleagues and they would eventually reach the acclimation stage where they would be able to work productively and "with a shared sense of purpose" with teams of health care workers [12].

In developing this framework, Daubman et al. further described the steps that could be taken to mitigate feelings of moral distress. Jacobs and Manfred suggested ways residency directors could help residents battle moral distress by encouraging directors to

- Have organized support groups, which would include an early residency ethics curriculum to help residents anticipate difficult ethical situations they might experience;
- Make certain that existing institution support structures such as crisis counseling programs, employee assistance programs, and grief counseling programs were publicized so that residents were aware of their existence;
- Encourage residents to seek assistance from hospital ethics, rationing, and/or palliative care teams;
- Create small group forums to facilitate collective sharing on difficult ethical cases, enhance communication, and address conflict management;
- Be flexible in assigning residents to electives or non-clinical training modules to allow time to process grief;

- Schedule residents on shifts to allow for call-outs or short-term leaves of absence. This will allow residents to reestablish existing support systems outside of residency [9].

As I covered in Chap. 1, moral distress and moral disengagement are known to adversely impact healthcare workers, including medical residents, and the care they provide to patients. Under the stress of a worldwide pandemic, the factors that led to both of these were especially prevalent. Medical residents found themselves in a position they would never have anticipated where their education was interrupted or had to be adapted, the hours they worked were long and stressful, and they faced constant policy changes as hospitals learned to cope with an unfamiliar and unanticipated situation. While more experienced clinicians were better able to adapt to the tensions and demands of COVID-19, those who were new to the field experienced burnout, which resulted in feelings of powerlessness, cynicism, and detachment from their work.

While conditions under COVID-19 were unusual, the issues faced by many healthcare workers during this time were similar to those generally found in healthcare and emphasized the need to understand the stressors that can impact healthcare workers' mental health.

However, along with Jacobs and Manfred's recommendations for residency directors to help residents stave off moral distress, there are also activities individuals can engage in to mitigate the physical and emotional demands of their jobs. Chapter 8 suggests practices medical residents can adopt to help them manage stress and the pressures of their residencies.

References

1. Jaqua E. Residency training in the COVID-19 pandemic: adaptation, exhaustion, opportunity. Reflective MedEd. 2021. https://reflectivemeded.org.
2. Laloo R, Karri RS, Wanigasooriya K, et al. The perceived global impact of the COVID-19 pandemic on doctors' medical and surgical training: an international survey. Int J Clin Pract. 2021;75(8):e14314. https://doi.org/10.1111/ijcp.14314.
3. Murphy B. Residency in a pandemic: how COVID-19 is affecting trainees. American Medical Association; 2020. https://www.ama-assn.org/medical-residents/medical-resident-wellness/residency-pandemic-how-covid-19-affecting-trainees.
4. Ferrel MN, Ryan JJ. The impact of COVID-19 on medical education. Cureus. 2020;12(3):e7492. https://doi.org/10.7759/cureus.7492.
5. Wilson CA, Metwally H, Heavner S, Kennedy AB, Britt TW. Chronicling moral distress among healthcare providers during the COVID-19 pandemic: a longitudinal analysis of mental health strain, burnout, and maladaptive coping behaviours. Int J Mental Health Nurs. 2022;31(1):111–27. https://doi.org/10.1111/inm.12942.
6. Wolf LA, Perhats C, Delao AM, Moon MD, Clark PR, Zavotsky KE. "It's a burden you carry": describing moral distress in emergency nursing. J Emerg Nurs. 2016;42(1):37–46. https://doi.org/10.1016/j.jen.2015.08.008.
7. Norman SB, Feingold JH, Kaye-Kauderer H, Kaplan CA, Hurtado A, Kachadourian L, Feder A, Murrough JW, Charney D, Southwick SM, Ripp J, Peccoralo L, Pietrzak RH. Moral dis-

tress in frontline healthcare workers in the initial epicenter of the COVID-19 pandemic in the United States: relationship to PTSD symptoms, burnout, and psychosocial functioning. Depress Anxiety. 2021;38(10):1007–17. https://doi.org/10.1002/da.23205.

8. Messner E, Parascando JA, La Gamma C, Bone C, Clebak KT, Riley TD. Effects of early COVID-19 restrictions on resident well-being and burnout. Fam Med. 2022;54(9):708–12. https://doi.org/10.22454/FamMed.2022.233405.

9. Jacobs B, Manfredi RA. Moral distress during COVID-19: residents in training are at high risk. AEM Educ Train. 2020;4(4):447–9. https://doi.org/10.1002/aet2.10488.

10. Dzeng E, Colaianni A, Roland M, Levine D, Kelly MP, Barclay S, Smith TJ. Moral distress among American physician trainees regarding futile treatments at the end of life: a qualitative study. J Gen Intern Med. 2016;31(1):93–9.

11. Senior J. The psychological trauma that awaits our doctors and nurses. New York Times; 2020. https://www.nytimes.com/2020/03/29/opinion/coronavirus-ventilators-rationing-triage.html.

12. Daubman B-R, Black L, Goodman A. Recognizing distress in the COVID-19 pandemic: lessons from global disaster response. J Hosp Med. 2020;15(11):696–8. https://doi.org/10.12788/jhm.3499.

13. Sims H, Alvarez C, Grant K, Walczak J, Cooper LA, Ibe CA. Frontline healthcare workers' experiences and challenges with in-person and remote work during the COVID-19 pandemic: a qualitative study. Front Public Health. 2022;20(10):983414.

14. Patterson JE, Edwards TM, Griffith JL, Wright S. Moral distress of medical family therapists and their physician colleagues during the transition to COVID-19. J Marital Fam Ther. 2020;47(2):289–303. https://doi.org/10.1111/jmft.12504.

Chapter 8
What Individuals Can Do

While Jacobs and Manfred have suggested ways directors can help healthcare workers and residents deal with stress on the job, it is also important that those working in the health fields find their own ways to manage the pressures caused by facing life and death situations, overwork, and interactions with administration. Much research is being applied to finding de-stressors that are effective in mitigating those effects.

Meditation and Mindfulness

Meditation is one practice that has been found to be helpful in managing stress. Behan defined meditation as "a formal practice that can calm the mind and enhance awareness of ourselves, our minds and our environment" and explained that, "over time, regular practice of mediation allows individuals to react to their environment and anything that arises in the course of their day with more calm and equanimity" [1]. This practice is especially useful for healthcare professionals who are overwhelmed, fearful, and under stress. Studies have shown a decrease in anxiety and stress in those who have meditated over a period of time [2].

La Torre et al. examined the effects of practicing mindfulness on healthcare workers and concluded that "mindfulness-based interventions (MBIs) … have emerged as unique approaches for effectively and comprehensively addressing a range of clinical and subclinical difficulties such as stress, chronic pain, anxiety, or recurrent depression" [3].

Joshi et al. studied the efficacy of transcendental meditation (TM), a "meditation practice in which individuals silently recite a single mantra (a sound that lacks meaning) without concentration or contemplation" for reducing stress on health care workers. They found those who practiced TM for 20 minutes twice a day for 3 months experienced significantly reduced effects of emotional exhaustion and burnout [4].

A. Ochasi, *The Challenged Resident*, https://doi.org/10.1007/978-3-031-71206-7_8

A study conducted by Shapiro et al. found health care professionals who participated in practicing mindfulness-based stress reduction (MBSR), a form of meditation meant to cultivate personal awareness and insight, reported, "decreased perceived stress and greater self-compassion" as well as decreased job burnout and increase in satisfaction with life [5].

Physical Relaxation Methods

In discussing the effectiveness of yoga and other mind-body meditation programs, Cocchiara et al. stated they "provide some innovative solutions, scientifically recognized as effective methods to enhance empathy, reduce stress and improve physical work-related issues in healthcare professionals," adding the clinical trials on the use of yoga and meditation have shown significant results in stress management and the reduction of burnout and in overall improvement of quality of life [6].

Zhang et al. suggested physical methods, such as yoga, massage therapy, and progressive muscle relaxation, could be helpful in mitigating healthcare workers' stress and burnout [7]. Results of a study undertaken with healthcare workers indicated "yoga and related exercises may be the most effective methods of stress reduction," explaining, "modulation of the autonomic nervous system appears to play a role, and studies have documented reductions in heart rate, blood pressure, and breath rate suggestive of reduced sympathetic and/or increased parasympathetic activity" [7]. Along with yoga, massage therapy was found to significantly reduce stress in healthcare workers.

La Torre et al. studied the effects of yoga practice on stress management and prevention of burnout among healthcare workers and found yoga helped decrease anxiety and long-term yoga practice mitigated aspects such as fear, weakness, and anger [3]. La Torre et al. also suggested both the practice of yoga and meditation could be incorporated into workplace health promotion in healthcare settings [3].

Creative Arts Therapy

Another practice found to be beneficial for individuals for relieving stress and burnout is creative arts therapy (CAT). One of the goals of CAT is to help people develop communication skills through the arts. This might be especially effective for healthcare workers who may not be able to express why they are stressed or for those who believe feeling stressed or burned out may be a weakness. According to Reed et al., "Arts-based encounters can be effective in reducing stress and burnout in health care workers, specifically increasing participants' self-esteem, reducing stress, stimulating personal growth, reducing work-related fatigue, improving communication and relationships, and promoting a sense of community at work" [8]. Creative arts therapy can include art therapy, music therapy, dance/movement therapy, and therapeutic writing, including keeping journals. The goal is to give healthcare workers who have experienced trauma and stress a vehicle through which they

> can bring authentic emotions to their experience and then use the resulting expression to communicate in visual, musical, written, or physical form. Participants may be able to confront, reflect on, and better cope with traumatic experiences by reconstructing meaning and developing transformative methods [8].

Moss et al., writing about the successfulness of creative arts therapy in relieving stress and burnout, discussed how work-related psychological stress increased during the COVID-19 pandemic. In implementing a CAT program where participants used art, photography, writing, and dance to depict and share their experiences, they found CAT was "associated with significant improvements in multiple measures of psychological distress including symptoms of anxiety, depression, posttraumatic stress disorder, and all three domains of burnout. Participants also had improvements in positive affect, and reductions in negative affect" [9].

Prayer

In discussing how incorporating self-care management can help nurses deal with stress and burnout, Nilsson suggested that prayer can help relieve the pressures associated with being in healthcare and cites the number of data that show "there is good reason to suppose that nursing professionals will greatly benefit from setting aside time each day for self-care practices which encourage self-reflection, freshen the spirit, and enable the continued administration of respectful, loving care" [10]. Nilsson described how one of the benefits of prayer includes "the ability to achieve emotional catharsis and/or spiritually cope with the pressures of tragic or painful" [10].

Norful et al., in studying the physical and psychological impact of stress during COVID-19, interviewed healthcare workers about the role of prayer in mitigating stress. One interviewee described how her unit incorporated spirituality to reduce stress:

> We created a prayer team. My boss implemented it. We pray before we start our shift. I also have a good support system at home. If I'm [working] and I get overwhelmed, I'll pick up the phone and call and pray over the phone. It's a strong support to keep me positive through a difficult time [11].

Wachholtz and Rogoff, while researching medical students' stress and burnout, found religion and spirituality can serve as protective factors against burnout. Their study showed medical students' personal spirituality helped them cope with the daily pressures and anxieties of their studies. In their conclusion, they stated,

> Students having higher levels of spiritual wellbeing and daily spiritual experiences described themselves as more satisfied with their life in general, while students with low scores on spiritual wellbeing and daily spiritual experiences had higher levels of psychological distress and burnout [12].

Studies of healthcare workers have shown that while during pre-COVID-19 over 60% percent of medical personnel experienced stress leading to burnout, [13] with the onset of the pandemic, numbers increased significantly, leading to concerns about the effect on patient care. As we've discussed, it should be incumbent upon hospitals and clinics to implement support and wellness measures to eliminate the root causes of stress among healthcare workers. However, it is also important that individuals find their own strategies to reduce their stress levels. Healthcare workers have the responsibility to care for patients and to deal with the pressures of the job. Lifewise, prioritizing their own wellbeing to stay healthy and satisfied with their work should be a paramount concern. Adopting strategies, such as meditation, yoga, exercise, and prayer, among other activities, can help reduce healthcare workers' stress levels and promote mental and emotional wellbeing.

References

1. Behan C. The benefits of meditation and mindfulness practices during times of crisis such as COVID-19. Ir J Psychol Med. 2020;37(4):256–8. https://doi.org/10.1017/ipm.2020.38.
2. Afonso RF, Kraft I, Aratanha MA, Kozasa EH. Neural correlates of meditation: a review of structural and functional MRI studies. Front Biosci. 2020;12(1):92–115. https://doi.org/10.2741/S542.
3. La Torre G, Raffone A, Peruzzo M, Calabrese L, Cocchiara RA, D'Egidio V, Leggieri PF, Dorelli B, Zaffina S, Mannocci A. Yoga and mindfulness as a tool for influencing affectivity, anxiety, mental health, and stress among healthcare workers: results of a single-arm clinical trial. J Clin Med. 2020;9(4):1037. https://doi.org/10.3390/jcm9041037.
4. Joshi SP, Wong A-K I, Brucker A, Ardito TA, Chow S-C, Vaishnavi S, Lee PJ. Efficacy of transcendental meditation to reduce stress among health care workers: a randomized clinical trial. JAMA Netw Open. 2022;5(9):e2231917. https://doi.org/10.1001/jamanetworkopen.2022.31917.
5. Shapiro SL, Astin JA, Bishop SR, Cordova M. Mindfulness-based stress reduction for health care professionals: results from a randomized trial. Int J Stress Manag. 2005;12(2):164–76. https://doi.org/10.1037/1072-5245.12.2.164.
6. Cocchiara RA, Dorelli B, Gholamalishahi S, Longo W, Musumeci E, Mannocci A, La Torre G. Tai Chi and workplace wellness for health care workers: a systematic review. Int J Environ Res Public Health. 2020;17(1):343. https://doi.org/10.3390/ijerph17010343.
7. Zhang M, Murphy B, Cabanilla A, Yidi C. Physical relaxation for occupational stress in healthcare workers: a systematic review and network meta-analysis of randomized controlled trials. J Occup Health. 2021;63(1):e12243. https://doi.org/10.1002/1348-9585.12243.
8. Reed K, Cochran KL, Edelblute A, Manzanares D, Sinn H, Henry M, Moss M. Creative arts therapy as a potential intervention to prevent burnout and build resilience in health care professionals. AACN Adv Crit Care. 2020;31(2):179–90.
9. Moss M, Edelblute A, Sinn H, Torres K, Forster J, Adams T, Morgan C, Henry M, Reed K. The effect of creative arts therapy on psychological distress in healthcare professionals. Am J Med. 2002;135(10):1255–62. https://doi.org/10.1016/j.amjmed.2022.04.016.
10. Nilsson H. Spiritual self-care management for nursing professionals: a holistic approach. J Holist Nurs. 2021;40(1):64–73. https://doi.org/10.1177/08980101211034341.
11. Norful AA, Rosenfeld A, Schroeder K, Travers JL, Aliyu S. Primary drivers and psychological manifestations of stress in frontline healthcare workforce during the initial COVID-19

outbreak in the United States. Gen Hosp Psychiatry. 2021;69:20–6. https://doi.org/10.1016/j.genhosppsych.2021.01.001.

12. Wachholtz A, Rogoff M. The relationship between spirituality and burnout among medical students. J Contemp Med Educ. 2013;1(2):83–91. https://doi.org/10.5455/jcme.20130104060612.

13. National Academies of Sciences, Engineering, and Medicine. Taking action against clinician burnout: a systems approach to professional well-being. The National Academies Press. 2019; https://doi.org/10.17226/25521.

Conclusion

The primary focus of this book was on how medical residents' experience of moral distress can lead to eventual moral disengagement, which can, in turn, impact patient care. As medical residents themselves pointed out in the interviews, feeling moral distress can stem from having to face, on a day-to-day basis, situations that are beyond their control. These include being left out of the decision-making process of patient treatment, unnecessary prolongation of life, and lack of supervisory support. As I argue, while the medical climate of healthcare organizations could have a positive effect on residents' experience, in fact, past studies have shown that, typically, the medical establishment often dismisses residents' concerns. Nor does it acknowledge that a negative environment can have biological, psychological, and stress-related consequences that ultimately lead to career dissatisfaction and ineffective patient care.

The COVID-19 pandemic only exacerbated these issues in the United States as it affected public health, education, industries, and employment. As I discussed in chapter 5, the pandemic also significantly impacted the medical field, including the education of medical residents in terms of curriculum changes, adoption of alternative education models, new innovations such as using computer based simulations, and receiving live or recorded lectures online. While COVID-19 put a strain on medical residents' wellness, and burnout became even more of a concern, many medical schools put certain support structures into place to mitigate the pressures residents were under. These structures, such as modifying work schedules during the pandemic and the development of support and solution-focused meetings, were thought to have a positive impact on the residents.

Stark et al. commented on policies put into place to support the physical and psychological wellbeing of residents during the pandemic stating, "Some of the most effective interventions included the construction of platforms to disseminate rapidly changing clinical information, improved access to psychological counseling services, increased mentorship opportunities, and augmented meal support" [1]. Lucey and Johnston suggested that over time COVID-19 will be "viewed as a

A. Ochasi, *The Challenged Resident*, https://doi.org/10.1007/978-3-031-71206-7

catalyst for the transformation of medical education." However, the focus of their work was on how "the physician workforce … will address the enduring competencies of professionalism, service, patients, and personal accountability, … embrace new competencies that are better suited to addressing today's health challenge" [2]. While their point is valid and the transformations necessary, what should be added to their vision is the wellbeing of residents as they go through their programs.

The pandemic can be said to have jolted our sense of consciousness within the medical field. One outcome has been the recognition that the traditional approach to education has to change. As noted, to ensure residents were able to cope physically and psychologically with the heavy demands of caring for patients during the pandemic in the face of shortages of equipment, long hours, and isolation, programs were implemented to aid in reducing medical personnel's moral distress and burnout. These programs proved to be effective.

On a practical basis, the pandemic brought to the fore the need for medical schools to adapt curriculums and new competencies relevant to today's health challenges. Whereas medical institutions might have been reluctant to change the medical education model before the pandemic, circumstances were such that there was no choice but to be flexible and innovative in education delivery. This same flexibility and innovation should be applied—or, in some cases, continued to be applied—to the psychological and physical wellbeing of medical residents. As schools and hospitals acknowledged the importance of helping medical professionals deal with the stress they were under during the height of the COVID-19 pandemic, it became apparent that residents benefited from programs directors implemented, from support groups to adjusting shifts to giving residents a voice in how the patients for which they were responsible were treated. Research has shown acknowledging and being proactive in confronting many of the stressors that medical residents face mitigates the risk of experiencing moral distress and moral disengagement, to the advantage of both future doctors and the patients who will rely on them.

The impetus for the original study and this book was to examine the relationship between moral distress and moral disengagement among U.S. medical residents and the residents' perception of the role of the ethical climate on moral distress and the propensity for moral disengagement. The challenge for the administration and leadership of health care institutions, especially residency directors, is recognizing the problem this phenomenon poses to residents and putting mechanisms in place to address it whenever it occurs. This is necessary for breaking the cycle of indifference that has dogged the issue of moral distress in residency programs. As we have seen, some of these changes took place in medical institutions during COVID-19. However, further work still needs to be undertaken to ensure the wellbeing of medical residents and to counteract the effects of moral distress. Not addressing the subject not only affects the residents and the care they provide to patients but also perpetuates the culture of inaction and denial of a critical issue in the medical establishment.

Appendix A: Moral Distress Physician Questionnaire (ADULT)

Moral distress occurs when professionals cannot carry out what they believe to be ethically appropriate actions because of internal or external constraints. The following situations occur in clinical practice. If you have experienced these situations, they may or may not have been morally distressing to you. Please indicate how frequently you experience each item described and how disturbing the experience is for you. If you have never experienced a particular situation, select "0" (never) for frequency. Even if you have not experienced a situation, please indicate how disturbed you **would** be if it occurred in your practice. Note that you will respond to each item by checking the appropriate column for two dimensions: *Frequency* **and** *Level of Disturbance*.

| | Frequency | | | | | Level of disturbance | | | | |
| | Never to very frequently | | | | | None to great extent | | | | |
	0	1	2	3	4	0	1	2	3	4
1. Provide less than optimal care due to pressures from administrators or insurers to reduce costs										
2. Witness healthcare providers giving "false hope" to the patient or family										
3. Follow the family's wishes to continue life support even though I believe it is not in the best interest of the patient										
4. Initiate extensive life-saving actions when I think they only prolong death										
5. Follow the family's request not to discuss death with a dying patient who asks about dying										
6. Feel pressure from others to order what I consider to be unnecessary tests and treatments										
7. Continue to participate in care for a hopelessly ill person who is being sustained on a ventilator, when no one will make a decision to withdraw support										

A. Ochasi, *The Challenged Resident*, https://doi.org/10.1007/978-3-031-71206-7

	Frequency					Level of disturbance				
	Never to very frequently					None to great extent				
	0	1	2	3	4	0	1		2	3	4
8. Avoid taking action when I learn that a physician or nurse colleague has made a medical error and does not report it										
9. Assist another physician who in my opinion is providing incompetent care										
10. Be required to care for patients I don't feel qualified to care for										
	Frequency					Level of disturbance				
	Never to very frequently					None to great extent				
	0	1	2	3	4	0	1	2	3	4
11. Let medical students perform painful procedures on patients solely to increase their skill										
12. Provide care that does not relieve the patient's suffering because I fear that increasing the dose of pain medication will cause death										
13. Request nurses or others not to discuss the patient's prognosis with the patient or family										
14. Increase the dose of sedatives/opiates for an unconscious patient that I believe could hasten the patient's death										
15. Take no action about an observed ethical issue because the involved staff member or someone in a position of authority requested that I do nothing										
16. Follow the family's wishes of the patient's care when I do not agree with them but do so because of fears of a lawsuit										
17. Work with nurses or other healthcare providers who are not as competent as the patient care requires										
18. Witness diminished patient care quality due to poor team communication										
19. Ignore situations in which patients have not been given adequate information to ensure informed consent										
20. Watch patient care suffer because of a lack of provider continuity										
21. Work with levels of nurse or other care provider staffing that I consider unsafe										
If there are other situations in which you have felt moral distress, please write them and score them here:										
[a.]										
[b.]										

Have you ever left or considered quitting a clinical position because of your moral distress with the way patient care was handled at your institution?

Appendix B: Moral Disengagement

Below are statements with which you may agree or disagree. Using the 1–7 scale below, indicate your agreement with each item by indicating that response for each statement.

Q.22 It is okay to spread rumors to defend those you care about.

- Strongly agree (1)
- Agree (2)
- Somewhat agree (3)
- Neither agree nor disagree (4)
- Somewhat disagree (5)
- Disagree (6)
- Strongly disagree (7)

Q.23 It is alright to lie to keep your friends out of trouble.

- Strongly agree (1)
- Agree (2)
- Somewhat agree (3)
- Neither agree nor disagree (4)
- Somewhat disagree (5)
- Disagree (6)
- Strongly disagree (7)

Q.24 Taking something without the owner's permission is okay, as long as you are just borrowing it.

- Strongly agree (1)
- Agree (2)
- Somewhat agree (3)
- Neither agree nor disagree (4)
- Somewhat disagree (5)

- Disagree (6)
- Strongly disagree (7)

Q.25 It is okay to gloss over certain facts to make your point.

- Strongly agree (1)
- Agree (2)
- Somewhat agree (3)
- Neither agree nor disagree (4)
- Somewhat disagree (5)
- Disagree (6)
- Strongly disagree (7)

Q.26 Considering the ways people grossly misrepresent themselves, it is hardly a sin (immoral) to inflate your own credentials a bit.

- Strongly agree (1)
- Agree (2)
- Somewhat agree (3)
- Neither agree nor disagree (4)
- Somewhat disagree (5)
- Disagree (6)
- Strongly disagree (7)

Q.27 Compared to other illegal things people do, taking something small from a store without paying for it isn't worth worrying about.

- Strongly agree (1)
- Agree (2)
- Somewhat agree (3)
- Neither agree nor disagree (4)
- Somewhat disagree (5)
- Disagree (6)
- Strongly disagree (7)

Q.28 People shouldn't be held accountable for doing questionable things when they were just doing what an authority figure told them to do.

- Strongly agree (1)
- Agree (2)
- Somewhat agree (3)
- Neither agree nor disagree (4)
- Somewhat disagree (5)
- Disagree (6)
- Strongly disagree (7)

Q.29 People cannot be blamed for misbehaving if their friends pressured them to do it.

- Strongly agree (1)
- Agree (2)
- Somewhat agree (3)
- Neither agree nor disagree (4)
- Somewhat disagree (5)
- Disagree (6)
- Strongly disagree (7)

Q.30 People can't be blamed for doing things that are technically wrong when all their friends are doing it.

- Strongly agree (1)
- Agree (2)
- Somewhat agree (3)
- Neither agree nor disagree (4)
- Somewhat disagree (5)
- Disagree (6)
- Strongly disagree (7)

Q.31 It is okay to tell a lie if the group agrees that it is the best way to handle the situation.

- Strongly agree (1)
- Agree (2)
- Somewhat agree (3)
- Neither agree nor disagree (4)
- Somewhat disagree (5)
- Disagree (6)
- Strongly disagree (7)

Q.32 Taking personal credit for ideas that were not your own is no big deal.

- Strongly agree (1)
- Agree (2)
- Somewhat agree (3)
- Neither agree nor disagree (4)
- Somewhat disagree (5)
- Disagree (6)
- Strongly disagree (7)

Q.33 Walking away from a store with some extra change doesn't cause any harm.

- Strongly agree (1)
- Agree (2)
- Somewhat agree (3)
- Neither agree nor disagree (4)

- Somewhat disagree (5)
- Disagree (6)
- Strongly disagree (7)

Q.34 Some people have to be treated roughly because they lack feelings that can be hurt.

- Strongly agree (1)
- Agree (2)
- Somewhat agree (3)
- Neither agree nor disagree (4)
- Somewhat disagree (5)
- Disagree (6)
- Strongly disagree (7)

Q.35 It is okay to treat badly somebody who is badly behaved.

- Strongly agree (1)
- Agree (2)
- Somewhat agree (3)
- Neither agree nor disagree (4)
- Somewhat disagree (5)
- Disagree (6)
- Strongly disagree (7)

Q.36 People who get mistreated have usually done something to bring it on themselves.

- Strongly agree (1)
- Agree (2)
- Somewhat agree (3)
- Neither agree nor disagree (4)
- Somewhat disagree (5)
- Disagree (6)
- Strongly disagree (7)

Q.37 If a business makes a billing mistake in your favor, it is okay not to tell them about it because it was their fault.

- Strongly agree (1)
- Agree (2)
- Somewhat agree (3)
- Neither agree nor disagree (4)
- Somewhat disagree (5)
- Disagree (6)
- Strongly disagree (7)

Appendix C: Ethical Climate Questionnaire

We would like to ask you some questions about the general climate in your hospital/health system. Please answer the following in terms of how it really is in your hospital/health system, not how you would prefer it to be. Please be as candid as possible; remember, all your responses will remain strictly anonymous. Please indicate whether you agree with each of the following statements about your hospital/health system. Please use the scale below and write the number which best represents your answer in the space next to each item. To what extent are the following statements true about your hospital/health system?

Strongly disagree	Disagree	Undecided	Agree	Strongly agree
1	2	3	4	5

Q.38 In this hospital/health system, people are mostly out for themselves.

Q.39 The major responsibility for people in this hospital/health system is to consider efficiency first.

Q.40 In this hospital/health system, people are expected to follow their own personal and moral beliefs.

Q.41 People are expected to do anything to further the hospital/health system's interests.

Q.42 In this hospital/health system, people look out for each other's good.

Q.43 There is no room for one's own personal morals or ethics in this hospital/health system.

Q.44 It is very important to strictly follow the hospital/health system's rules and procedures here.

Q.45 Work is considered substandard only when it hurts the hospital/health system's interests.

Q.46 Each person in this hospital/health system decides for himself what is right and wrong.

Q.47 In this hospital/health system, people protect their own interest above other considerations.

© The Editor(s) (if applicable) and The Author(s), under exclusive license to
Springer Nature Switzerland AG 2024
A. Ochasi, *The Challenged Resident*, https://doi.org/10.1007/978-3-031-71206-7

Q.48 The most important consideration in this hospital/health system is each person's sense of right and wrong.

Q.49 The most important concern is the good of all the people in the hospital/health system.

Q.50 The first consideration is whether a decision violates any law.

Q.51 People are expected to comply with the law and professional standards over and above other considerations.

Q.52 Everyone is expected to stick by hospital/health system rules and procedures.

Q.53 In this hospital/health system, our major concern is always what is best for the other person.

Q.54 People are concerned with the hospital/health system's interests to the exclusion of personal interests.

Q.55 Successful people in this hospital/health system go by the book.

Q.56 The most efficient way is always the right way, in this hospital/health system.

Q.57 In this hospital/health system, people are expected to strictly follow legal or professional standards.

Q.58 Our major consideration is what is best for everyone in the hospital/health system.

Q.59 In this hospital/health system, people are guided by their own personal ethics.

Q.60 Successful people in this hospital/health system strictly obey the organization's policies.

Q.61 In this hospital/health system, the law or ethical code regarding theft is a major consideration.

Q.62 In this hospital/health system, each person is expected, above all, to work efficiently.

Q.63 It is expected that you will always do what is right for the customer and public.

Please answer a few questions about yourself.

Q.64 Are you an intern, resident, or fellow?

- Intern
- Resident
- Fellow

Q.65 What is your year of residency?

- Internship/PGY-1
- PGY-2
- PGY-3
- PGY-4
- PGY-5
- PGY-6
- PGY-7
- Not Applicable

Q.66 What is your year of fellowship?

- First year
- Second year
- Third year
- Fourth year
- Fifth year
- Sixth year
- Seventh year
- Not applicable

Q.67 What is your specialty in residency?

- Family Practice
- Internal Medicine
- Emergency Medicine
- Emergency Medicine and Family Practice
- General Surgery
- Cardiology
- Pediatrics
- Pulmonology
- Critical Care
- Anesthesiology
- Obstetrics/Gynecology
- Psychiatry
- Radiology
- Radiation Oncology
- Gastroenterology
- Orthopedic Surgery
- Neurosurgery
- Geriatrics
- Endocrinology
- Dermatology
- Hospitalist
- Not Applicable

Q.68 What is your specialty in fellowship?

- Family Practice
- Internal Medicine
- Emergency Medicine
- Emergency Medicine and Family Practice
- General Surgery
- Cardiology
- Pediatrics
- Pulmonology
- Critical Care
- Anesthesiology
- Obstetrics/Gynecology

- Psychiatry
- Radiology
- Radiation Oncology
- Gastroenterology
- Orthopedic Surgery
- Neurosurgery
- Geriatrics
- Endocrinology
- Dermatology
- Hospitalist
- Not Applicable

Q.69 What is your gender?

- Male (4)
- Female (5)

Q.70 How would you rate your level of ethics education from medical school to residency/fellowship?

- None
- Low
- Moderate
- High

Q.71 What is the highest level of education you have completed?

- Grammar school (4)
- High school or equivalent (5)
- Vocational/technical school (6)
- Some college (7)
- Bachelor's degree (8)
- Master's degree (9)
- Doctoral degree (10)
- Professional degree (MD, JD, etc.) (11)
- Other (please specify) (12) _____

Q.72 What is your marital status?

- Single, never married (1)
- Married or domestic partnership (2)
- Widowed (3)
- Divorced (4)
- Separated (5)
- Would rather not say (6)

Q.73 Which of the following best describes your race or ethnicity?

- African American (Black) (1)
- Caucasian (White) (2)

- Asian/Pacific Islander (3)
- Latino(a)/Hispanic (4)
- Middle Eastern (5)
- Multiracial (6)
- Other (Please specify) (7) _____
- Would rather not say (8)

Q.74 What is your age?

- 18–24 years old (1)
- 25–34 years old (2)
- 35–44 years old (3)
- 45–54 years old (4)
- 55–64 years old (5)
- 65–74 years old (6)

Appendix D: Interview Questions (Qualitative Phase)

1. Can you describe some incidents you encountered during your residency that caused you moral distress?
2. How would you name the emotions you experienced? Are some of these experiences more intense than others and how would you describe the frequency of the experiences?
3. Describe the coping mechanisms you deployed to deal with moral distress during your residency.
4. In hospitals, some patients are dubbed "frequent fliers" because they are in and out of the hospitals. Some residents believe that these patients do not follow the advice of clinicians in making the necessary lifestyle changes to improve their health outcomes. How do you feel about such patients?
5. How would you describe the ethical climate of your hospital?
6. How would you characterize the support from your supervisors and hospital administration when you experienced moral distress?

References

1. Stark N, Hayirli T, Bhanja A, Kerrissey M, Hardy J, Peabody C. Unprecedented training: experience of residents during the COVID-19 pandemic. Ann Emerg Med. 2022;79(5):5. https://doi.org/10.1016/j.annemergmed.2022.01.022.
2. Lucey CR, Johnston SC. The transformational effects of COVID-19 on medical education. JAMA. 2020;324(11):1033–4. https://doi.org/10.1001/jama.2020.14136.